The Memory System of the Brain

The Memory System of the Brain

BY

J. Z. Young

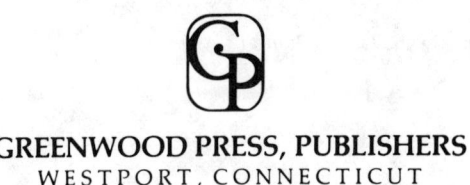

GREENWOOD PRESS, PUBLISHERS
WESTPORT, CONNECTICUT

Library of Congress Cataloging-in-Publication Data

Young, J. Z. (John Zachary), 1907–
    The memory system of the brain.

    Reprint. Originally published: Berkeley and Los
Angeles : University of California Press, 1966.
    Bibliography: p.
    1. Memory--Physiological aspects. 2. Brain.
I. Title.
QP406.Y68 1986   153.1   85-30577
ISBN 0-313-25096-0 (lib. bdg. : alk. paper)

Reprinted with the permission of University of California Press

Reprinted in 1986 by Greenwood Press, Inc.
88 Post Road West, Westport, Connecticut 06881

Printed in the United States of America

10 9 8 7 6 5 4 3 2 1

Preface

These Hitchcock Lectures, delivered at the University of California, Berkeley, California, in November, 1964, are now published approximately in the form in which they were given. This has the disadvantage that the somewhat personal style may seem out of place in print, but perhaps there are compensating advantages. The view of nervous activities presented here is a personal one. It has been arrived at with the assistance of the work of many colleagues, but they do not by any means always agree with my conclusions. To all of them I should like to express my warmest thanks. Brian Boycott devised and carried out many of the early experiments with the octopus. Mrs. Marion Nixon helped with the more recent ones and Vernon Barber and George Savage assisted in the preparation of this book. Mrs. Jane Astafiev prepared many of the illustrations. Mr. G. Sommerhoff helped at many points with criticism of my ideas, as have others with whom I have been lucky enough to work, including N. S. Sutherland, E. G. Gray, W. R. A. Muntz, N. J. Mackintosh, J. Mackintosh, M. J. Wells and J. Wells. I am most grateful to all of them.

It is a pleasure also to thank the various individuals and organisations who have given their co-operation.

First, Dr. P. Dohrn and the staff of the Zoological Sta-
tion at Naples, without whom the work on the octopus could not have been done. Mr. A. Packard has been
especially helpful in many ways. Mr. J. Armstrong
supervised much of the work in London on the structure of the brain, and Miss P. Stephens carried out the
extensive histological preparations. The work has been
aided financially by the Nuffield Foundation, and more
recently by the European Office of the United States
Office of Aerospace Research, to whom we are most
grateful.

The structures in the octopus brain and the phenomena of learning shown by the animal have stimulated me to develop a system of ideas about cerebral
coding and memory, which are incorporated in the
recent book, *A Model of the Brain*. The present work
is in the main a summary of this, but such systems develop with each reformulation. There is much here
that has not been published elsewhere, especially on
the touch learning system and the origin of memory.

Finally, it is a great pleasure to thank the University of California and all those in Berkeley and Los
Angeles who welcomed me for the delivery of the lectures. Professor W. J. Asling, Professor T. H. Bullock,
and many others combined to give me some idea of the
greatness of the University of California.

J. Z. Young, M.A., D.Sc., F.R.S.

Department of Anatomy
University College, London
February, 1965

Contents

CHAPTER ONE

The Brain as the Computer
of a Homeostat

Explanation in Biology

Probably we should all agree that the question "How do brains work?" is important and that it would be a good thing to know the answer, but would there be agreement on the form the answer might take? The brain is an exceedingly complicated system and our language and powers of understanding are but weak. In what sense therefore can we expect to be able to say, "I understand the brain"?

In the last analysis, the most severe criterion by which we judge our understanding of a system is our ability to take it to pieces and then put it together again, or make one like it. This might seem to be an absurdly ambitious criterion to apply to the brain, though it can be argued that in some respects we are already moving toward this end. We are beginning to come within sight of the power to make simple living things. It will be a long step from that to making a complex brain, but who is to say that this goal will not be achieved? In the meantime perhaps we should be more humble. We are so far from a complete understanding of the brain that we must not yet expect to be able to see a complete picture, but must be content for the present with what I shall call a model of the brain. We shall try to build this model from various sources. The present chapter presents various facts about the basic components of the nervous system. These are necessary before we can attack the much more interesting and difficult question of how to think about the way in which these components are assembled to make a whole brain.

For that synthesis, when we come to it, we may rely mainly on two sources. First, the facts of the organisation of the relatively simple brain and memory system of the octopus provide us with a model with which to approach the complex human brain. Second, to organise this information we shall explore how far it is possible to use the terminology of computer science. Computers are machines that perform some of the actions of brains. Apart from their great practical value they equip us with a language with which we can describe and discuss brains.

Throughout human history there have been repeated cycles of discovery. A substitute is invented to assist an activity previously performed only by human beings or animals, for example engines that assist the labour of man's hands. The basic sciences evolve alongside the development of such artifacts, studying the principles of operation of the tools and providing a language by which better machines can be produced. These are, in turn, applied to produce further new knowledge. To make a machine work properly it is necessary to understand its principles thoroughly. Every engineer knows this and every biologist should learn it from him. With the aid of the more exact language, biology is much better able than before to "explain" the living process for which the substitute was invented. This cycle has been repeated over and over again. For example, "energy," a concept originally applied only to living things, has been greatly refined and can now be used to give a vastly better understanding of biology.

Thus one group of meanings given to the word "explanation" as applied to living activities is certainly connected with the capacity to devise machines that assist in these activities. One of the most exciting advances of our age is the development of machines that help with some functions previously performed only by brains. But computers and automatic control systems do more than this. They actually imitate some of the features of living things as a whole. To some extent they are self-maintaining systems or homeostats, the name invented by W. B. Cannon of Harvard, the Hitchcock Lecturer in 1941 (Cannon, 1932). No man-made system is yet able to maintain itself over a prolonged period, nevertheless, from the humble gas oven or icebox to the guided missile or automatic factory, we now have many examples of machines in which *control* is exercised. These have become possible because of the development in this century, especially over the last twenty years, of a scientific study of the function that we call "control," previously a property attributed only to living systems. In particular there has been a great advance in understanding the principles of control through feedback systems, giving rise to what have been called directive correlations, for example servomechanisms (Sommerhoff, 1950). The language and the mathematics developed for the study of artifacts are available to biologists in their investigations of the organs that exercise control in the living body, especially the deoxyribosenucleotides of the nuclei, and the networks of nerve-cell fibres in the brain.

I propose to try to show to what extent we may be said to understand the brain in the terms that are used by engineers in their studies of communication, of computation, and of control. But my point of view throughout is that of a biologist, indicating the connections with these other methods of description rather than pursuing them in detail. I shall be using examples from machines to form a model that may help in understanding the brain.

To simplify, I shall, for the most part, deal not with the human brain but with that of the octopus, which is complicated enough to be interesting but not too complicated for us to begin to understand it. Moreover, the very unfamiliarity of the animal, in its behaviour and in the parts of its brain, forces us to think hard about such matters as motivation and memory. I shall also use the word "model" in yet another sense, saying that the brain contains a model of the animal's world, that indeed each species of animal or plant in a sense "models" or represents the world around it. Of course each species has receptors that detect changes only in a limited number of features that are relevant to its life. It can be said to represent the outside world only in respect of these features.

The Maintenance of Homeostasis
by Selection of Responses

One of the first questions to ask if we are to understand any machine is "What is it for?" As regards the brain, the answer may be phrased as follows. Brains are the computers of homeostats and the essence of homeostats is that they maintain a steady state. Put in another way, the most important fact about living things is that they remain alive. Curiously enough, this is not always the central theme in discussions of living processes, though perhaps it should be. It may immediately be objected that a principal characteristic of organisms is that they die, and although the point is irrelevant we must deal with it. Living things maintain an astonishing stability. The mammals are older than the Rocky Mountains. But this survival is made possible only by a special device, which in a sense evades the problem. Permanent self-maintenance seems to be a logical impossibility. Every sort of machine has defects and these can be repaired only by other special repair machines and so on ad infinitum. "What repairs the repairer that repairs the repairer . . . ?" Living things escape this regress by the subtle means that we ordinarily call reproduction. They do not attempt indefinite repair. At intervals they discard the whole machine, *keeping only the instructions by means of which it is rebuilt*. These instructions are then combined (in sexual organisms) with the set that built a slightly different machine, and with the combined instructions a new model that is slightly different from either of the old ones is produced.

Thus living systems do not avoid the paradox. They are not truly self-maintaining systems; they maintain an approximately constant organisation only by repeatedly changing into something slightly different. This change is, of course, evolution, which thus appears as the long-term aspect of homeostasis. This shows the significance of the life cycle of birth, growth, and death. The entity that is preserved is not the individual but something greater, which goes on when each individual dies. The processes of reproduction and of evolution are direct continuations of the processes of control of bodily functions that we ordinarily deal with as the physiology of homeostasis.

All control consists in selection of the right response from a repertoire of possible actions of the system. Organisms remain alive by selecting at each moment of time the appropriate response. In the processes that we ordinarily call "physiological" we see how the animal selects the right values, say of its heart rate, to suit the circumstances. In evolution there is similarly selection of the right instructions to allow survival. The changes of evolution are in effect long-term physiological adjustments, long-term homeostasis.

The continuance of life for short term or long is thus dependent on selection of the response that is appropriate to whatever circumstances occur. We may define "information," at least for our present purposes, as the feature of any change in the communication channels of a homeostat that allows selection of an appropriate response. For adequate selection the basic instructions (or construction) of the homeostat must obviously correspond to the events that are likely to occur in the environment. It may be said to *represent* the environment, in the literal sense that it re-presents to it the actions that are needed for survival.

The wide capacity to perform efficient actions is one of the most striking characteristics of living things. Even the simple system of bacteria has a range of adaptability that seems almost miraculous. These capacities are the end product of a storage of information about the environment that has been going on for a long time, perhaps 3,000 million years. We are beginning to be able to speculate about how the capacity to form large sets of possible actions arose. It may well be connected with the power of the carbon atom to form series of homologous compounds. However this may be, the capacity to remain alive clearly depends upon the presence of a variety of possible responses and their suitability for the environment.

The Nervous System as Selector of Responses

This rapid examination of some principles of biology has, I hope, brought us nearer to a view of some of the aspects of homeostats that are relevant to an understanding of the brain. The brain, as the computer, plays a key part in selecting the responses that are made by the animal. Recognition of this factor of choice between alternatives is the central feature that makes it possible for us to understand the function of the brain.

The body has a large set of effectors by which to act upon the environment in order to ensure survival. For example, all the muscles are arranged in pairs, flexors

and extensors, across the joints. By enumeration of the
pairs it should be possible to estimate the number of
actions that might be undertaken, bearing in mind that
not all combinations are equally probable. In this way
an exact and quantitative study of behaviour might be
attempted. It is essential to appreciate the implications
of the fact that actions are produced by repeated selection between pairs of alternatives. The information
that implements this selection is embodied in the brain
in a form not entirely different from that of a digital
computer, which also deals in selection between alternatives. But at this stage we must beware of over-
simplification. The choices between alternatives are
not usually made in a strictly logical or even sequen-
tial manner. The processes in the organism reflect the
changes in the environment and in turn influence
these. The question, therefore, whether the brain functions more like a digital machine or an analogue machine is not easily answered.

Nerve Fibres as Communication Channels

Certainly, the nerve impulses, the signals conducted in
peripheral nerves, are of an all-or-nothing digital nature. The researches of many investigators from Keith
Lucas and Adrian to Gasser, Joseph Erlanger (also a
former Hitchcock Professor), and a host of others
throughout the world have established that the operation of the appropriate effector organ, say a muscle or
gland, depends upon passage along the correct channel of trains of signals, the nerve impulses, which are
all essentially alike. The frequency in the channel de-

termines the degree of action, but usually carries no other information. The code is not one with several items in each channel, like a Morse code. Codification consists in selecting the right ones among a large number of channels, and the sensory or receptor channels function similarly.

These are very crude statements and much more could be written on the subject, but it is clear that in a multichannel system the number of channels is one of the most important variables and some figures may be useful. The numbers of fibres leading to the effector organs are moderate. Eccles and Sherrington found 233 to the soleus muscle of the cat. There are about 120,000 somatic motor fibres all together in a cat. They are more numerous in the nerves that control delicate movements, for instance of the eyes, than in those that regulate powerful actions of the limbs. An octopus has about 110,000 motor fibres leaving its brain (excluding those to the blood vessels and chromatophores).

The receptor channels are more numerous. In man there are unknown numbers of peripheral receptors (more than 100×10^6 in each eye) and about 3×10^6 afferent channels on each side leading to the brain. One million of them come from the eye, but only 30,000 from the ear. The octopus has a total of 8×10^6 peripheral receptors (other than in the eyes), but they transmit to the brain by only some 40,000 channels. Each eye of the octopus has 20×10^6 receptors and the same number of channels to the optic lobe.

If we had more facts about the numbers and sizes of cells and fibres we might understand the nervous system better. The numbers are often large, sometimes very large. But this is not simply a matter of ensuring redundancy, for some parts operate with far fewer channels. Each of the stellar nerves of the mantle of a squid has only one enormous fibre (up to a millimetre in diameter) though there are other smaller fibres with it.

Speed of conduction is one of the variables of the fibres; the larger fibres conduct faster. Diameter increase alone is a very inefficient way of obtaining fast conduction, since the velocity increases only with the square root of diameter, as theory predicts.[1] Fast conduction in the channels of the homeostat is obviously an advantage in a fast-moving world, and special means of obtaining it are found in the interrupted myelin sheaths that allow a saltatory conduction in vertebrates and probably in prawns and shrimps. Only these special devices for increasing velocity make it possible for a fast moving animal to have numerous channels. The nerves of the human arm contain hundreds of thousands of fibres, which would obviously be impossible if each had to be half a millimetre in diameter.

The small fibres are as interesting as the large. Why are there so many of them? Sometimes it must be a matter of economy. Each of the 20,000,000 fibres in the optic nerves of the octopus is about 1μ in diam-

---

[1] We have recently confirmed this by a study of conduction velocities in fibres of the octopus, cuttlefish, and squid. Fibres of similar diameters in the three species conduct at similar rates and dimensional factors seem to preponderate. The smallest fibres studied were about 2μ and conducted at <1 m/sec; the largest 500μ, at 23 m/sec. The best estimate over the whole range is that the velocity follows $D^{0.57}$ (Burrows *et al.*, 1965).

eter. If they were only ten times larger they would oc-
cupy an area greater than that of the entire surface of
the animal. But economy can hardly be the only factor,
for often there are numerous small fibres, although
the functions to be performed seem to require little
resolution. Thus, although the whole musculature of
the head and eyes of an octopus is controlled by a mere
3,000 fibres, the nerves that control the salivary glands
contain nearly a million fibres. This large number
surely cannot mean an equally large power of differ-
ential response by the gland cells.

Nerve Cells and Synapses as Computers

The great difference between the nervous system and
digital machines is in the large number of points at
which computation is made. As von Neumann (1958),
among others, has pointed out, the artificial computer
makes its decisions in only a few organs and makes
them very fast and in a highly regulated and logical order. The nervous system has many computing organs,
for each nerve cell acts as such, and they are relatively
slow and unreliable.

Computers work with localised memory stores, each
point in which carries a single item of information,
whose significance is determined by the fact that it has
a precise "address." It is still an open question whether
nervous systems contain any such highly addressed
memory system. There must, in man at least, be a record of individual occurrences, and means for consulting that record. Yet much evidence shows that the neural memory system is distributed rather than localised.

There are dangers in using the language invented for computers, with their localised memories, for nervous systems, which are certainly rather different. Some scientists think that it would be wiser to avoid the computer language in neurology. Here we shall accept the risk of inappropriateness for the sake of the increased possibility of communication and indeed for the actual stimulus to investigation that the computer analogy provides. But the danger remains, and we should be continually aware that the analogy between brains and computers may be misleading.

And yet, the difference may not be so great as it might seem. It is true that the particular qualities of the digital computer are its speed and its generality. It can do anything if it is properly programmed to do it, whereas the nervous system is not a general computer; it can do only certain things, but it can take the data about these things direct from the environment. It is a special-purpose computer carrying its programme in the coded instructions of its DNA and the constructions to which they give rise. Yet, in spite of these differences, the operations that it controls are fundamentally those of selection from a code of possible alternative actions.

The numbers of nerve cells give us some measure of computing power. There are $1 - 2 \times 10^{10}$ of them in man and $1 - 2 \times 10^8$ in an octopus brain, but there are also 3×10^8 in the octopus' arms. This animal really does "think with its hands." We say that the nerve cells act as computers because the nerve impulses must be initiated afresh in them. Each nerve fibre conducts in an all-or-nothing manner, probably without decrement to its very ends. But where these ends come into contact with the receptive dendrites of the next cell in the chain the individual impulses do *not* invariably pass on. Only if impulses arrive suitably distributed in time along one fibre or distributed in space over the endings on the dendrites does the cell emit a signal (or change its rate of signalling). The cell and the points at which it receives synaptic junctions from other fibres thus serve to add the effects of these presynaptic fibres. There is also subtraction, since some of them inhibit the setting up of impulses by the postsynaptic cell.

A great deal is known about the mode of operation of the synaptic junctions, where one nerve cell stimulates another, which, collectively, are thus the computers at which decisions are made whether a nerve cell shall send out a signal. Yet our knowledge has been limited by the difficulty of obtaining a view of the whole set of synapses on a cell with the microscope, or a record of their individual actions by microelectrodes. The terminal buttons that constitute the synapse were not even known for certain to exist throughout the cerebral cortex until nine years ago, when we found that they can be revealed by a method that stains their mitochondria (Wyckoff and Young, 1956). They do not show up readily with the classical silver methods that reveal these "boutons" in the spinal cord and elsewhere. The failure of cortical boutons to stain is probably due to the fact that they do not contain neurofibrils (though these may appear during degeneration). The density of boutons on motor cells of the spinal cord reaches 20 per $100\mu^2$; according to estimates of the area of these cells, there are some 30,000 boutons per cell (Wyckoff and Young, 1956; Aitken and Bridger, 1961). In the cerebral cortex they are much smaller than the boutons on spinal cord cells, and there may be 10,000 of them on a large pyramidal cell, but the surface areas of these are not known accurately, and the number of boutons per cell may be much greater.

Electron microscopy has told us a great deal about the detailed structure of synapses, including those of the cerebral cortex. They always show vesicles on the pre-synaptic side and differentiations of various sorts in the region of contact (Gray, 1964). Unfortunately we do not understand the molecular biology of these thickenings and therefore cannot assess their significance. We do not know whether the "truly synaptic" or transmitting portions of the boutons are the thickenings where vesicles are aggregated. Further, we have little secure evidence about the differences between boutons that are excitatory and those that are inhibitory. Some of the latter may be placed in positions where they can block the arrival of impulses along the presynaptic fibres. Endings that could do this have been seen by electron microscopy in the retina, spinal cord, and some centres in *Octopus* (Kidd, 1962; Gray, 1962).

The electron microscope has shown us much detail of synapses, but so far we cannot fully interpret it. It has not been possible to add much to our quantitative knowledge of synapses by electron microscopy. We do not know how much of the surface of cells and dendrites is covered by the transmitter regions. The space between the presynaptic and the postsynaptic membranes is still a controversial subject, and there are few data about the proportions of surface that are covered by the glia (the supporting and filling tissue of the nervous system; Kuffler and Potter, 1964). Even worse, for most parts of the system we have no idea whether one incoming fibre sends boutons to one or to many cells, nor whether all the boutons from one presynaptic source are grouped together or whether they are mixed with boutons from other fibres.

I mention these enormous gaps in knowledge not out of pessimism but in the hope of stimulating the development of methods that will enable us to answer these quantitative anatomical questions. We must know the answers if we are to understand the nervous system, yet most investigators prefer to follow the current vogue of placing electrodes within cell bodies that can be entered, or identifying the chemical molecules that are extractable from centrifugates. I do not wish to decry neurological studies of these or any other sorts, but to urge that perhaps *they should be guided more by what logic tells us we need to know, and less by the techniques found suitable in other disciplines.* The nervous system is a multichannel network. The first requirement for understanding it is to know its connectivity. Those who work out the connections have been the major pioneers of neurology. This appears very clearly from the work of C. S. Sherrington and Ramon y Cajal, who, together with many others, have established the model of the brain that we still use. Both men based their work on concepts of connectivity and Sherrington, the physiological experimenter par excellence, made his own anatomical and histological enquiries.

The study of cerebral connectivity is still in its infancy and demands the greatest powers that science can produce. To choose four fields as examples: (1) The development of machine methods for counting and measuring cells and fibres is obviously essential to supply the data relevant to a multichannel system. (2) The staining methods of Golgi and Cajal provide marvellously informative details of connectivity but we have no idea of the underlying physical and chemical principles of the stains. (3) The electron microscope provides resolution amply sufficient to see large molecules, but we have minimal information about what has been done to them by fixation. (4) We cannot even reconstruct whole neurons from electron micrographs.

The Organisation of the Nervous System

This survey of some aspects of knowledge about the nervous system may serve to introduce the means that we hope to use in building a model of the brain, which is perhaps the farthest we can go toward understanding it. We must know the nature of its units—neurons, nerve fibres, axons, dendrites, synapses—and have examples of how they function. Then we must know a good deal about the connectivity and especially the principles upon which it is based.

The sources of information with which the nervous system operates may be divided into three classes. First, there are receptors for signalling information from the outside world. Second, there are receptors that detect the departures from required levels of operation of the various systems within the body and send signals that indicate what is needed for self-maintenance. These two sorts of signals provide the information on which selection of appropriate responses is based. Third, the homeostat needs information about the results of its actions—whether these have been satisfactory for self-maintenance or destructive to the organism. Receptors that signal "pain" or "taste" are typical examples. In simpler nervous systems these receptors operate reflex actions, such as feeding or withdrawal, and in such systems the instructions as to which action is to be taken depend upon the inherited connectivity. But in higher nervous systems the instructions are supplemented by information stored in the memory about the results of previous actions of the animal. The signals of results thus acquire the further function of teaching the memory store.

The Memory of the Nervous System

At the present time we are especially interested in the nature of the neural memory, and it is important to try to see its place in the whole system. We shall not understand it by thinking of its chemistry alone, any more than we should learn how information is stored in a book by studying the chemistry of ink. We shall advance in our study of memory only when we recognise that the brain is the computer of a homeostat and that the memory provides part of the information by which the homeostat selects correct responses.

We must be careful about the use of the word "memory." It will here be limited, as by an engineer, to the unit within which a record is stored. The record itself will be called a representation within the memory. An early task is to try to find the code in which the record is stored. We must, as it were, learn the language that is used in the writing in the brain. Recently there have been very great advances in understanding the hereditary material since biochemists realised that they must search for codes. They looked for them and found them in the DNA. Moreover, some workers have found it desirable to pursue the analogy to great lengths, looking for words and punctuation of the genetic language, systems for reading-in to the record and reading-out from it and even for the turning of pages.

Curiously, there has been relatively little of the equivalent search in the study of memory in the brain. Many biologists still find such analogies distasteful, even whimsical. Yet there is nothing strange in using the terminology of artificial aids to communication and memory, such as writing, as a means for speaking about the brain. This process of making artifacts and then borrowing their terminology back into biology has been a recurring process through the ages. Physiologists have no hesitation in using the concepts of volts and amperes in talking about nerve impulses, yet some of them are reluctant to speak of the impulses as "signals in a code." There is much to be done to clear up misunderstanding about the status of analogies and other forms of words in science. The historian and the logician can both help us here.

In the investigation of memory in the brain a logical experimental program with a thoughtful strategy is especially necessary because the concepts of "language" and "representation" are not familiar to all sci-

entists. We shall not find the memory change by prob-
ing with microelectrodes or by whirling bits of brain
in centrifuges unless we have such a strategy.

We may begin with the proposition that each animal's memory, if it is to assist in selecting adequate responses, must contain some "representation" of the
world in which it lives. This is a much stronger term
than to say that the brain contains an engram, for we
can use the analogy of "representation," for example
by writing, to guide us as to what sort of entity to look
for in the brain. Books are written with letters selected
from a pre-established alphabet. The next chapter de-
scribes the search that we have made for the fount, as
it were, from which letters are selected to print the
writing in the brain of the octopus. Some progress has
been made toward recognising them, in the forms of
the dendritic trees of certain cells. If this is right, we
can go farther and suggest how they are selected to
make the representation or model, as we may call it,
in the brain. By such a procedure we have been led
to look in the appropriate places for the changes
that constitute learning and have found there certain
small cells and certain types of synapse.

We have not found the nature of learning, but have
produced a rather coherent if somewhat childish picture of the whole process. This picture may seem so
unsophisticated as to be laughable, but the truth is often simple, at least in its general outlines. It is surprising how many living processes have been found to have
quite detailed similarity to simple mechanical processes. Life does involve many complications, but it is
the general outlines that we need here. Given these,

there will be many brains willing and able to fill in the complicated details.

We are sadly lacking in important data about the scheme of operation that will be suggested for the octopus brain, especially from microelectrodes and chemical procedures. The suggestions made here will almost certainly prove to be wrong in many respects, but I doubt whether we can be wholly wrong in our interpretation of how the various lobes of the octopus brain are used to write a record in the memory. As we have gradually traced the connectivity within this brain, it has revealed, with a curious inevitability, the basis of its logic, and perhaps the logic of all nervous systems (though they may not be all alike). The various lobes of the octopus brain are visible and distinct entities, arranged in a regular manner, and with a discernible order. They have differing types of neurons, which are readily stainable. The characteristics of the neurons and the fibre patterns of each lobe can, in some degree, be related to their places in the logical system. Moreover, the whole set of four lobes is repeated twice over. One set is associated with the visual memory; the other, with only minor differences, with the tactile memory. The approximate seats of the two actual records have been found and each can be removed separately without influencing the other.

The "centres" that we are talking about are undoubtedly really there and are distinct, although in life they may co-operate to some extent in ways that have not yet been revealed. The analysis can hardly be wholly wrong even if still some way from being right.

We may be wrong in holding that the representations are made by selection from an alphabet. It would be interesting to consider whether all representations are made with the use of pre-arranged codes. I should be inclined to say that they are. Like any agent in the process of information transfer, the representational nature of a physical event is defined by the fact that when this event occurs in the communication channels of an appropriate homeostat it elicits the selection of responses that are "correct" for homeostasis. This presupposes the existence of the type of pre-arranged correspondence that constitutes the definition of a code.

A further possibility is that we cannot usefully speak of the brain as containing a representation of the environment at all. Many who have been concerned with the problem of the adaptiveness of living activities have tried to deal with them without such language as I am using (Sommerhoff, 1950). It can even be argued that the brain does not have what can properly be called a memory in the computer sense, because it learns by changing its network and does not carry records of individual events. This objection surely falls because, in man at least, single particular events *can* be recalled and there must thus be a record of them. If it seems not to be so in other animals, this may be the result of our method of testing. Perhaps running animals in mazes is not the best way of finding out about the series of selections by which records are written in their brains. Of course it does not follow that the record of a "single event" is localised only at one place. In a multichannel system the record may be carried by changes at many points. Removal of some of them by injury or surgery may weaken the reliability with which the engram can control behaviour.

Whether the approach suggested here is invalidated by these or other criticisms will be shown by whether it leads toward the discovery of the nature of neural memory. I feel that it has led me further toward this end than did consideration of "adaptation" alone, although I have always been strongly interested in adaptation. But that concept is without much power until it is reinforced by consideration of sets of possibilities among which selection can be made.

The Octopus as an Experimental Animal

If we are to break the code of the brain it will be desirable to find a system that answers readily when we ask it such questions as whether object A is more similar to object B or to object C (e.g., Is a triangle more like a square or a circle?). From the responses of an animal that answers well we can discover what types of discrimination can be made and hence perhaps by what mechanism classification and discrimination are carried out. *Octopus vulgaris* is a very valuable subject in these respects. Much has been found out about the animal's visual powers by Boycott, Sutherland, Muntz, Mackintosh, Maldonado, and others. Its powers of discrimination by touch and chemical sense have been tested by Mr. and Mrs. Wells. The animal lives among the rocks, often hidden in a crevice, and comes out to attack objects moving in its visual field. The attack on an unfamiliar object is slow and cautious. If the object

written we must first search for the code set and then for the method of selection from it by the effects of pleasure and pain signals.

To obtain an understanding of the alphabet we must investigate the animal's capacity to learn to discriminate between formed stimuli. The octopus is a suitable animal for such experiments. It can learn to discriminate forms by sight or by touch. The memory stores for the two types of receptor are in separate parts of the brain. Each store is accompanied by four auxiliary lobes.

CHAPTER TWO

Breaking the Code
of the Brain

The Visual Code of the Octopus

The position we have arrived at is that brains are special-purpose computers designed to operate each in its own environment. If this is correct we should expect to find that each type has receptors and computing equipment appropriate only to its needs. This clue is so commonplace that we tend not to recognise its value, especially for studies of the brain. During the processes of evolution a large range of variants of brain design has appeared, constituting, as it were, a series of experiments whose results we can study and make use of in our attempts to understand the brain.

This type of approach is particularly helpful if we are looking for the language or alphabet of the brain. One of the classical procedures of cryptographers is to guess what the signals may be about, and thus to "break the code." Indeed, concealment of the subject matter is the intractable problem in military encoding. The matters that are likely to be under discussion by soldiers, sailors, or airmen can be guessed rather easily, however they may try to disguise them. Similarly it is not very difficult, by simple observation of the needs and actions of animals, to make hypotheses in regard to the features of the world that are of greatest interest to them. This step must be taken if we are to use studies with microscope and microelectrode to break the code of the brain.

Some progress has been made in analysis of the attributes of visual situations that can be distinguished by the octopus. Unfortunately, these studies are not based upon the behaviour of the animals in the sea, for of this almost nothing is known. In laboratory experiments Sutherland (1957) found that the animals are able to distinguish vertical from horizontal rectangles but not between oblique rectangles set at right angles. He suggested that their system of shape recognition depends at least in part on estimating the extent of outline in vertical and horizontal directions and taking a ratio between them. The animals discriminate poorly between figures that do not differ in vertical and horizontal extent, (e.g., square and circle). Conversely they make what seem to us erroneous decisions when they are presented with some figures. Thus animals trained to attack a square but not a horizontal rectangle, when shown a vertical rectangle treat it like the square. For the octopus system this is not the error that it seems to us. The ratio of horizontal extent to the area is 1.0 for the square and 2.2 for the horizontal rectangle, but only 0.4 for the vertical rectangle, which is, so to speak, more square than a square by this system.

Vertical and horizontal extents are not the only

aspects that are measured. Other suggestions have been made by Deutsch (1960, *a* and *b*) and by Dodwell (1957, 1961) to explain the experimental findings. Sutherland and Mackintosh (1964) have put forward evidence that in rats various parameters may be measured and that there is an initial process of "switching in" by which the system selects the parameter that it has learned will allow discrimination in a given situation.

Classifying by Orientated Dendrite Fields

The evidence that horizontal and vertical extents are of special importance agrees with some striking facts about the arrangement of the visual system. In the retina the sensitive elements are arranged in a rectangular array with the axes horizontal and vertical, as the head of the animal is normally held under the influence of the statocyst. The pupil is a horizontal slit. Projection from the retina to the optic lobe is through a remarkable nerve-fibre chiasma, which inverts the pattern of distribution in the dorsal-ventral plane alone (fig. 3). Whatever this may mean, it shows that the system demands the maintenance of particular spatial relations between the visual field and the optic lobe elements. Other visual systems also show this feature: the projections from the eye to the tectum opticum of fishes or amphibia, or to the thalamus and cerebral cortex of mammals, maintain the retinal topology. The optic chiasms in the mid-line of vertebrates may have a function of re-inverting the retinal image as does the "unilateral" chiasma of cephalopods (see Young, 1962 c). In the bee and other arthropods there is also a system ensuring re-inversion of the retinal information on each side of the body.

Within the optic lobe of an octopus the fibres end in a plexiform zone that has remarkable similarities to the nervous part of the retina of vertebrates (figs. 1 and 2).There are outer and inner layers of amacrine cells. These are neurons with no single axon, but a bush of short processes ending within the plexiform zone, where they spread to varying extents (fig. 3). The retinal cells have connections with these amacrine cells, whose significance is obscure. Perhaps they are concerned with lateral inhibition and hence with increasing the contrast of contours. This may also be the function of the efferent fibres, many of which proceed from the plexiform zone to end in the retina (fig. 3).

The retinal fibres pass on, ending in the deeper part of the plexiform zone, where layers of fibres spread in the tangential plane. These are the dendrites of cells lying deeper in the lobes, the next link in the neuronal chain (fig. 3). Many of these dendrite fields are ovals, with their axes often in the horizontal plane. The fibres of many cells together thus form a grid, orientated in the vertical and horizontal planes (figs. 4 and 5). It was suggested, following Sutherland's experiments, that these fields may detect contours, especially in the horizontal direction (Sutherland, 1963; Young, 1960 a). There was no microelectrode evidence on this point in the octopus, nor is there yet. But Hubel and Wiesel (1959, 1962, 1963, 1965), in their observations on the visual fields of cells of the visual cortex of the cat, have found that each cell "looks at" an oval visual field, of-

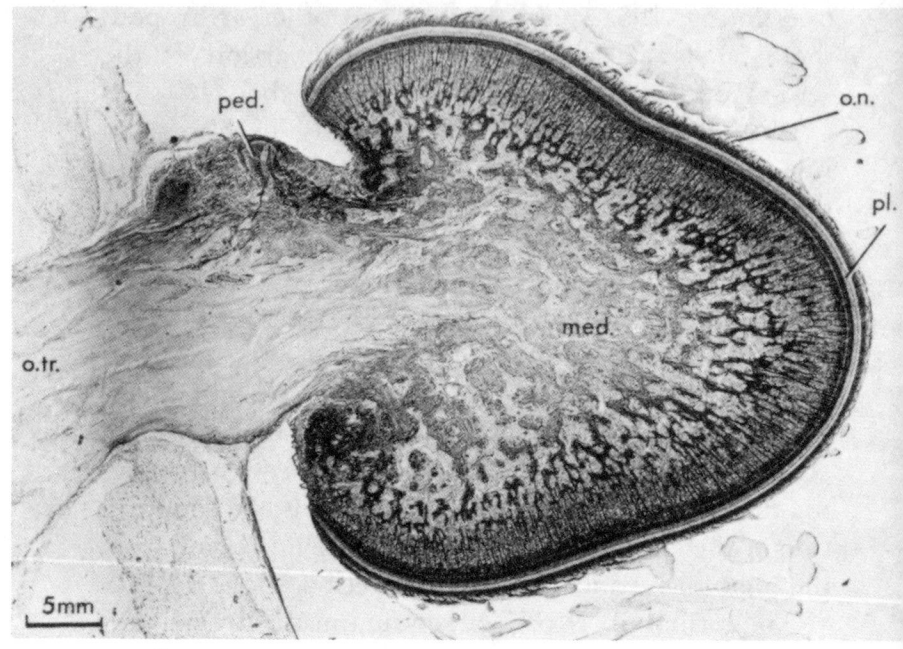

Fig. 1. Sagittal section of optic lobe of *Octopus*. med., medulla of optic lobe; o.n., optic nerve fibres (from retina); o.tr., optic tract (fibres to and from rest of brain); ped., peduncle lobe; pl., plexiform layer. (Young, 1962*b*)

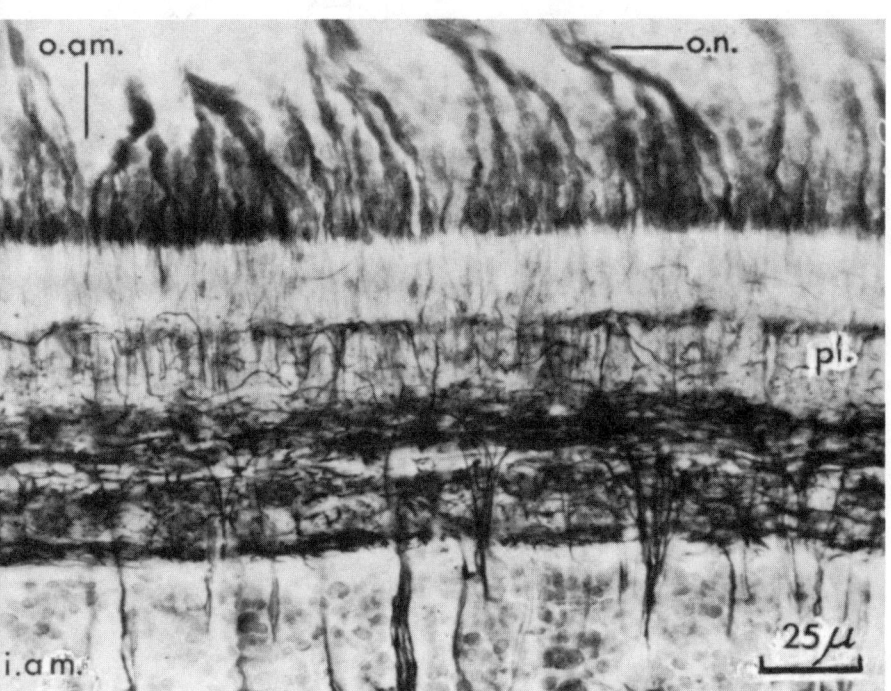

FIG. 2. Sagittal section of optic lobe of *Octopus*. i.am., inner layer of amacrine cells; o.am., outer layer of amacrine cells; o.n., optic nerve fibres (from retina); pl., plexiform layer. (Young, 1962*b*)

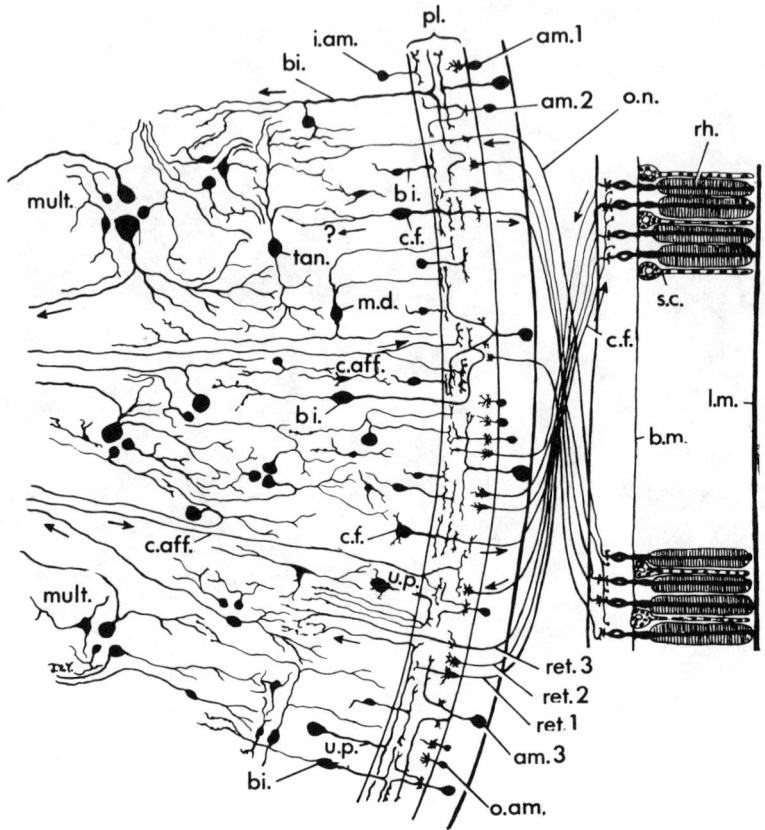

FIG. 3. Composite diagram of connections of neurons of optic lobe of *Octopus* as revealed by Golgi stain. am. 1–3, amacrine cells of outer granule cell layer; b.m., basal membrane; bi., bipolar cell; c.f., centrifugal fibre; c.aff., afferent fibre to plexiform layer from central regions; i.am., amacrine cell of inner granule cell layer; l.m., limiting membrane; m.d., cell with many dendrites proceeding outward; mult., small multipolar cell; o.am., amacrine cell of outer granule cell layer; o.n., optic nerves; pl., plexiform zone; ret. 1–3, retinal nerve fibres of three types; rh., rhabdome; s.c., supporting cell; tan., tangential cell of outer medulla; u.p., unipolar cell with a fibre running to plexiform zone and axons returning from this. (Young, 1962,*b*)

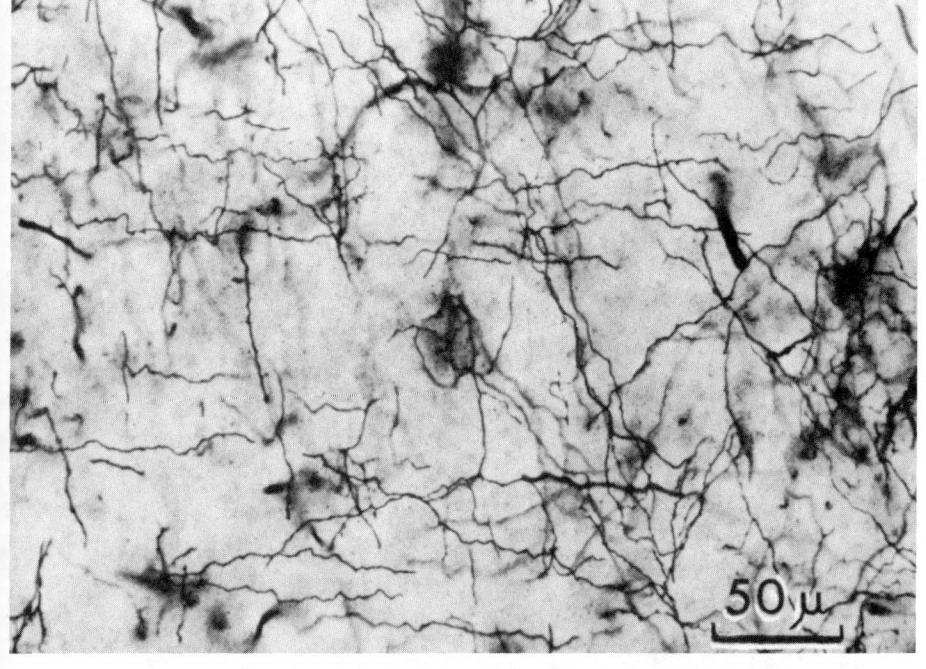

FIG. 4. Plexiform zone of optic lobe of *Octopus* seen in a section tangential to surface, showing dendrites running mainly in two directions, at right angles. Golgi stain.

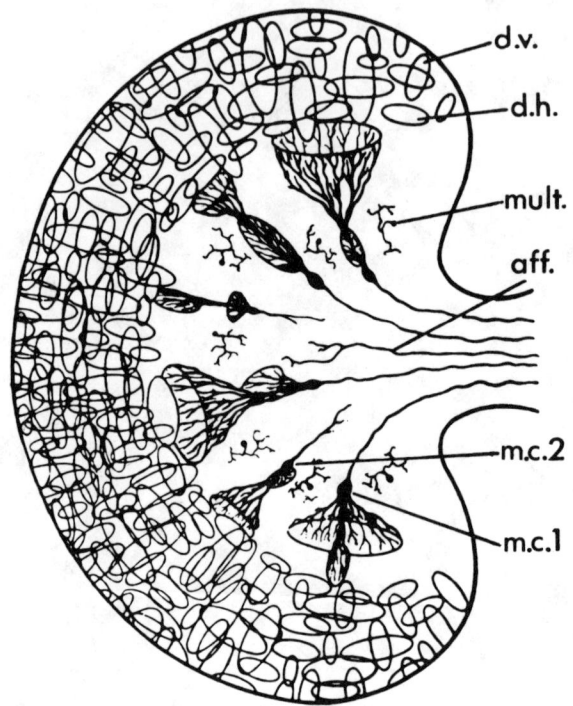

FIG. 5. Schematic diagram of arrangement of orientated dendrite fields of bipolar cells in optic lobe of *Octopus*. Some fields run vertically (d.v.), others horizontally (d.h.) Cells of medulla (m.c.1, m.c.2) with dendrites at different levels and in different orientations. aff., afferent fibres; mult., small multipolar cell. ⟨Young, 1960*a*⟩

ten with an inhibitory centre and an excitatory sur-
round or the reverse. Indeed, each such cell may
operate as a detector of contour with a particular orientation, exactly as postulated above for the optic lobe.
There are "simple" cells stimulated by illumination
only of a highly specific field and "complex" ones that
respond when illuminated by an area or edge with a
particular orientation lying anywhere within their
field. Thus some cells act as detectors for edges, dark
bars, or illuminated slits. In the octopus there is
certainly a preferential dendritic orientation of the
fields, as the appearance of the grid shows. Unfortunately, whole single fields can be picked out only oc-
casionally with the microscope, and the details of their
shapes remain to be studied. Some fields are very large,
more than half a millimetre across, corresponding to a
large angle in the visual field. In many fields the long
axis is horizontal, with several branches at right angles.

Hubel and Wiesel have not been able to study
enough cells with microelectrodes to decide whether
preferred orientations exist. However, Colonnier
(1964) has studied the organisation of the visual cortex as seen in Golgi preparations cut in the tangential
plane (figs. 6 and 7). He found many oval fields, as well
as round ones, belonging to both pyramidal and stellate cells. These may be the features that determine the
visual fields found by Hubel and Wiesel. Colonnier
found distinct signs of preferential organisation in the
visual cortex of the cat, with especially large numbers
of fibres in the directions that correspond to the vertical and horizontal planes of the visual field. Moreover,
he found orientated fields also in the cortex of the rat
and the monkey.

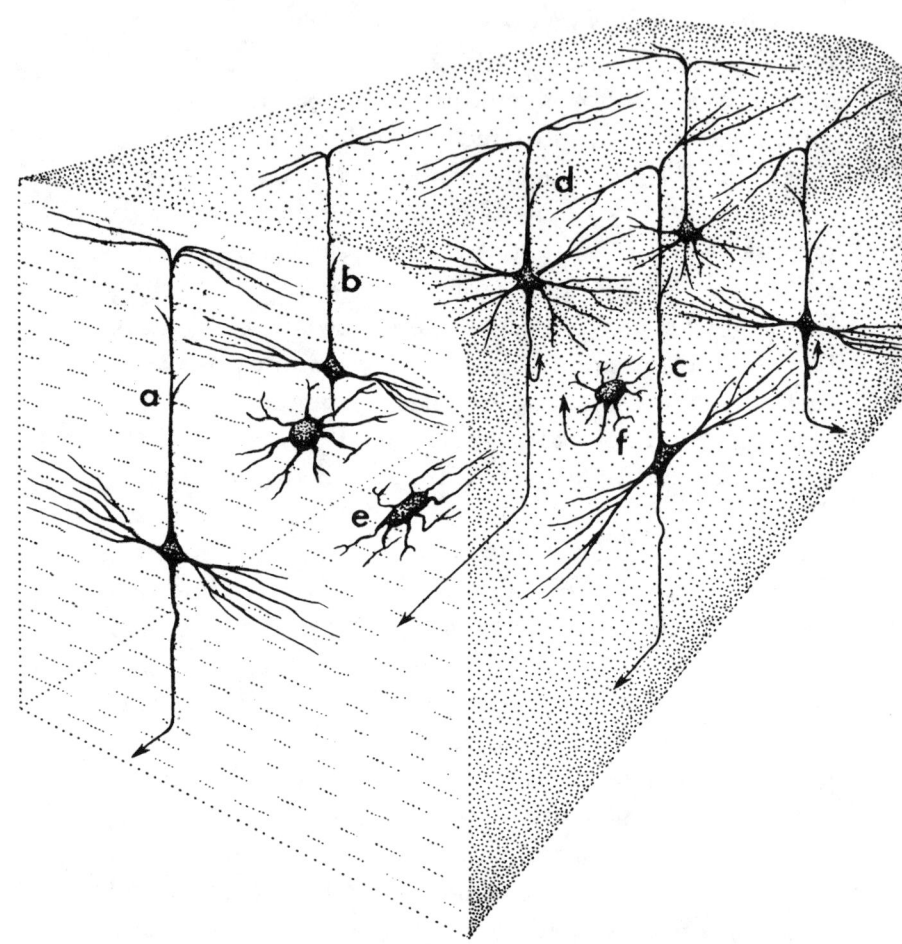

Fig. 6. Diagram of direction of spread of dendritic fields in visual cortex of cat (after Colonnier, 1964). Pyramidal cell *a* has apical and basal dendrite fields orientated in same (transverse) direction; *b* has its basal field transverse, apical longitudinal (anteroposterior). In *c* both are longitudinal. In *d*, basal field is cruciform; *e* is a stellate cell with an elongated field; *f* has a spherical field. Only some of the axons and their collaterals are shown.

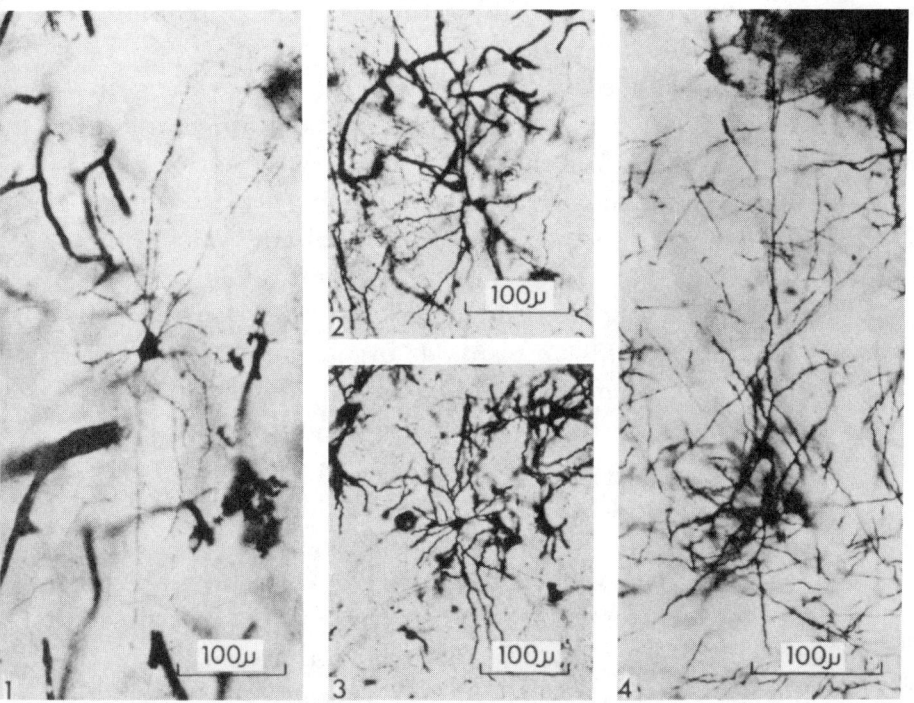

Fig. 7. Cells from visual cortex of cat seen in a section cut tangential to surface and showing elongated dendrite fields. 1. Basal dendrites and a pyramidal cell in layer VI. 2. Apical dendrites in layer I. 3. Basal dendrites of pyramidal cells in layers II and III. 4. Basal dendrites of pyramidal cell in layer IV. (Colonnier, 1964)

A striking result of these studies of the organisation of dendrites has been the discovery that individual dendrites run approximately straight for very long distances. We have heard much about the brain as a "random" system, but there is much that is not random about these dendrites; they must be highly determined at some stage in their growth. Hubel and Wiesel find that the fields have a similar orientation throughout each column of cells in the cortex. Other parts of the cerebral cortex have a similar organisation. In the somatic sensory cortex of the cat and the monkey the cells of a given vertical column respond to stimulation either of a particular area of skin or of deeper tissues such as a joint (Mountcastle, 1957; Powell and Mountcastle, 1959).

Sholl (1956) showed that there is an immense overlap between dendrite fields; each large pyramidal cell may share its field with up to 4,000 others. Any incoming fibre may connect with some among 5,000 cortical cells, spread through a volume of 0.1 mm^3. The possibilities of interaction between columns of cells responding to different orientations are therefore very large. Moreover, for pyramidal cells there is the possibility of different orientations of the apical and the basal dendrites. These features, together with the orientations of the dendrites of the short-axon stellate cells, would allow for a variety of combinations sufficient to explain even the subtle discriminations of shapes by man.

Learning as the Inhibition of Unwanted Pathways

To make the suggestion more explicit, we need a hypothesis that shows specifically how such cells could operate to provide the alphabet of the nervous system. The requirement seems to be that each classificatory cell shall be able to produce two (or more) outputs, leading to alternative actions. When the situation for which the cell encodes occurs in the visual field, one of these outputs is given and an action follows, say an attack on the object in the field. The detector systems for signalling results record the beneficial or prejudicial consequences of this action and these signals must then so alter the channels that the appropriate one is more likely to be used when the same situation occurs again.

Such a system has been postulated for the optic lobe of the octopus in figure 8. The classifying cells communicate each with two cells that may be called "memory cells," leading to channels for attack or retreat. The signals of results (e.g., taste or pain) arrive at the appropriate memory cells and, through collaterals of these, they pass to the opposite channel, which they inhibit. Learning consists in making this inhibition long-lasting, by changes (to be discussed later) which probably involve the small cells that are abundant in such centres (p. 93).

It should be made clear that only some of the components of this scheme of connections have been actually identified in the optic lobes. Cells that could act as classifying cells are there and they have axons with several branches among the cell islands nearer the cen-

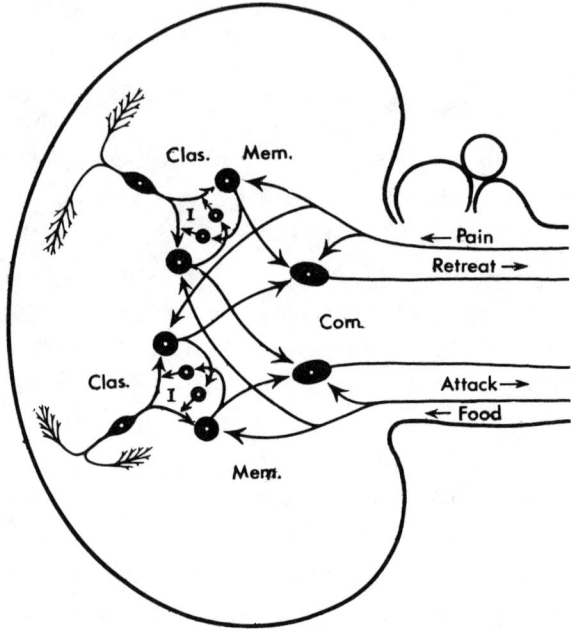

FIG. 8. A possible mode of functioning of the memory system in the optic lobes of *Octopus*. The shape of the object seen by the eye is analysed by dendritic fields of classifying cells (Clas.) in terms of horizontal and vertical extents. The information is passed to memory cells (Mem.), which, in the naïve state, pass on to command or motor cells (Com.) the signal to attack.

If the attack succeeds in securing food, fibres signalling this result activate the memory cells, increasing the excitability of those promoting attack in that situation. This may be achieved by the activation of small inhibitory cells (I), which, in this case, will prevent firing of memory cells whose output is to the motor cells governing retreat.

If the attack is punished, the memory cells receive a pain input; those cells governing retreat are activated, and in turn activate the inhibitory cells that suppress the tendency of the other memory cells to promote attack. (Young, 1964*a*) tre of the lobe. Here are cells with spreading dendritic branches, which may correspond to memory cells. These are accompanied by small multipolar cells, which may be the agents of inhibition, but the details of how all are connected have not yet been discerned in the complex tangle of fibres. In the islands nearest the optic tract are very large neurons that almost certainly initiate movements, since these can be elicited by electrical stimulation of this region, but not from other parts of the lobe.

The position is therefore that the components can be identified but their connections only in part. We can say only that the system *may* function approximately as suggested. The module of figure 8 has been made to include the two alternative possibilities, because an octopus can be trained to give either of two responses when a particular figure appears. Some experiments suggest, however, that in the initial situation the two outputs are not equally probable, that the tendency to attack is greater. Indeed, it is possible that the simplest learning systems had only a single outlet, the alternative being whether it should be open or closed.

The essence of the module is a group of cells specialised to alter the probability of the use of the channel (s) leading from a classifying cell. The alteration could be an increase or a decrease in any particular channel. If the change is complete it constitutes the storage of a single bit or item of information. It records whether stimulation of the given classifying cell was followed by results good or bad for the organism. This system for storing a single bit of information may perhaps be the unit we are looking for. Since the

Hitchcock Lectures were delivered, it has been suggested that it be called a mnemon (Young, 1965 *a*).[1]

If the system functions approximately as indicated, then, on any one occasion of seeing, only a limited number of the classifying cells will be stimulated, though the number may be extended to allow for generalisation (e.g., to the opposite eye; see p. 44). It is assumed that the inappropriate channels from the cells stimulated are fully closed by the signals of results arriving at the learning system, and that they do not reopen. Learning is thus complete for the cells stimulated on each presentation. The familiar slow development of the evidence of learning consists in the accumulation of enough trained cells to ensure a consistent response. Animals in their natural life may learn more rapidly than under the artificial conditions with which we test them in the laboratory. That human beings remember single occasions is obvious enough. The apparent slowness of learning in childhood may indicate that considerable time is required for the accumulation of a sufficient number of trained cells, appropriately interconnected to perform certain tasks.

The Model in the Brain

The various mnemons record which responses to each type of circumstance are likely to be good for the organism. The classifying cells at many levels are pre-

---

[1] Dr. A. Cherkin has kindly shown me his manuscript, suggesting that memory consists of units called mnemons (*Proc. Nat. Acad. Sci.* 55, Jan. 1966). He postulated these to account for gradations in the memory of chickens anaesthetised at various times after learning. The present hypothesis attempts to give a physical realisation of Cherkin's mnemons.

sumably able to record information in this way. Hubel and Wiesel have shown that there are cells able to respond to what they have called simple, complex, and hypercomplex features of the visual world.

So we can imagine a hierarchy of mnemons, constituting what may be called a model in the brain. This formulation or analogy was first used, I think, by Kenneth Craik of Cambridge in 1943, who was one of the earliest to develop ideas of the applications of control theory in biology and psychology. It is now possible to make the conception much more specific. A model is a representation. It is often made by selection and assembly of pieces from a set. What the brain learns must represent features of the world. Now it seems likely that this representation is made by selection among a set of cells, specified by their dendritic field systems.

The conception of a model often implies that the model works, and can be used to test possibilities by simulation, as a toy that is yet a tool. This is obviously true of the working model in our brains. Its value is primarily in enabling us to test out the probable consequences of various lines of action "in our heads" and then to decide what is likely to be the best course of action.

Representations in codes are used in homeostats for transmitting, storing, or manipulating the information by which self-maintenance is ensured, and this is exactly what the model in the brain does. Included in the concept of a model is that of the abstraction of the essentials of a situation, giving the expectation that perfectly forecastable and desirable results will follow from the use of a given model. This is the sense embodied in the use of the word "model" for a dress by a fashion designer, or for her mannequins by their admirers.

Without insisting too much on what is after all only one among many possible ways of speaking, we may thus find it reasonably helpful to say that as learning proceeds a model is built in the brain. Such a formulation stimulates us to look further for the elements of which the model is composed, for the method by which it is assembled, and how it is used. These are aspects of the anatomy and physiology of the nervous system that have not been sufficiently studied. The terminology of representation of the outside world by building a model in the brain will be justified if it leads to fruitful investigations and discoveries.

Transfer of Representations

If the dendritic fields of the cells of the optic lobes function as has been suggested, various problems of learning must be faced. If the change during learning consists in modification of the output from the cells that are stimulated, how do we account for transfer and generalisation of learning? There are very good opportunities for the study of transfer across the midline, since an octopus ordinarily uses one eye at a time and can be trained by figures shown exclusively in one visual field. Muntz (1961) has done this very successfully, showing that there is transfer and that it survives after removal of the optic lobe of the trained side. He investigated the commissures by which transfer takes place. For this transfer to occur the commissural system must include specific connections between classifying cells with similar field orientations on the two sides. This may seem to require a rather high degree of specificity in embryological development. However, since the discoveries by Sperry (see review by Gaze, 1960) and others of the high degree of specific connection in the vertebrate visual system, we should not be surprised to find that this is present to a relatively modest degree in the octopus. Interest in specific connections within the nervous system has revived in recent years, but there are still only a few who investigate the development of specificity.

The basic learning system suggested above requires a fairly high degree of specific built-in connections. The taste fibres must make connection with the pathways for attack and the pain fibres for retreat, but we are so used to seeing animals and men making the correct response (eating what is good and avoiding what is dangerous) that we have ceased to wonder at it. Animals do not commonly perform biologically absurd actions such as damaging their own tissues or starving to death in the midst of plenty. The systems of motivation and reward have become so subtle in man that they do sometimes produce deviations from behaviour that tend to preserve the individual (or even the race). These aberrations are part of the price that we pay for the advantages conferred in other ways by our elaborate and largely self-taught system of instructions. But most of us have enough specifically connected detectors of results to provide a reasonably high probability of survival (though pathological exceptions occur).

The classifying cells with two possible outputs in our scheme (fig. 8) obviously require specific connections to ensure opposite results from their two outputs. The collateral branches of the cells that have been called memory cells must have specific connections with small cells associated with the opposite pathway. To produce the learning system a fairly elaborate hereditary mechanism is required. But a memory can be a very valuable acquisition for a species, and under suitable circumstances there would be strong selection pressure to develop even a highly detailed morphogenetic mechanism for it. As we shall see in the last chapter, specific reciprocal connections are common in so-called reflex organisations that do not learn. To use a fashionable phrase, such systems are pre-adapted to evolve a memory mechanism.

Generalisation

The capacity for generalisation in the memory has also been studied in the octopus. When an animal has learned a specific discrimination it usually continues to perform correctly even when the situation is changed. For example, after learning to discriminate between white horizontal and vertical rectangles an animal may discriminate more or less correctly between black horizontal and vertical ovals. Many aspects of generalisation can be treated within our hypotheses by supposing that the dendritic fields that we have postulated as detectors are not rigidly restricted in their sensitivity and can be activated by situations that approximately resemble those that have been learned. If this is so, there must be limits to generalisation, and common sense tells us that this is true. We have investigated the limits for size generalisation in *Octopus* (Parriss and Young, 1962). As in other species, an octopus that has learned a discrimination between objects of one size can usually perform it also for larger sizes and to a lesser extent for smaller sizes. To investigate the capacity for generalisation more closely, we must avoid the obvious difficulty that an animal in moving about normally sees objects at a variety of retinal sizes. Octopuses are very convenient for such study because they can be made to remain in their homes. We accordingly trained them by giving rewards or shocks as soon as they began to move toward the figures, before they left the home, thus ensuring that they saw each figure only at one retinal size.

The capacity of these octopuses with limited movement to identify correctly the orientation of figures of other sizes was found to be much less than that of octopuses that were allowed to move toward the shapes and hence saw the figures at a range of retinal sizes (fig. 9). The capacity for generalisation in the animals with the smaller visual experience was more limited.

This suggests that no true process of generalisation really exists. What we call by that name may be the result only of the great variety of experience that active learning homeostats such as ourselves acquire over the years. The selecting of the responses that are likely to be most appropriate to the stimulation of the classifying cells of a given type proceeds continually—presumably until the whole fount of them is used up, if that stage is ever reached.

Reversal

Another problem is to show that the system suggested will account for reversal of the direction of learning.

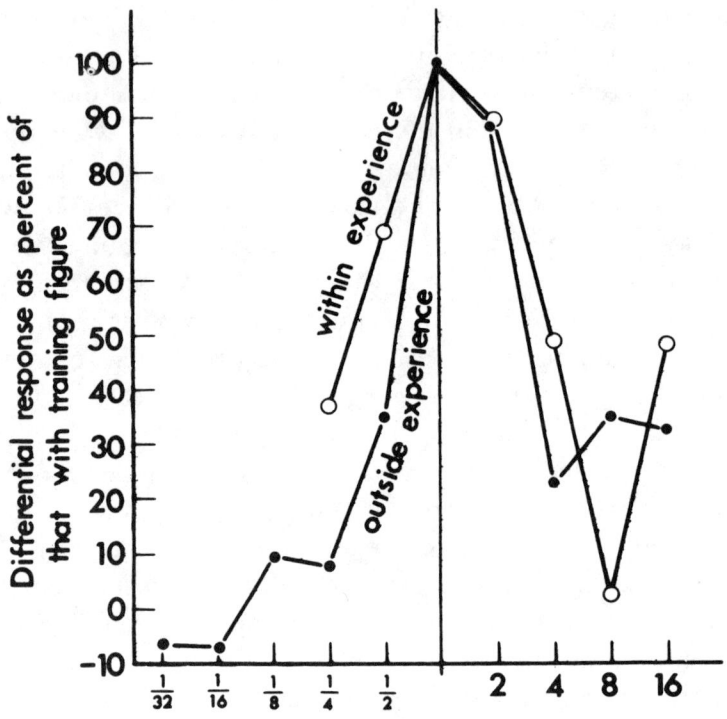

FIG. 9. Limits of size generalisation by *Octopus*. Accuracy of recognition during testing with vertical and horizontal rectangles of various sizes is expressed as a percentage of the accuracy with the figures used in training. Open circles, results for figures within the animal's experience during training. Solid circles, results with figures of sizes never seen during training; with these there is much less transfer, especially to smaller figures. (Parriss and Young, 1962)

After reversal the octopus continues for a considerable time to show signs of the original direction of training. The new representation in the memory is additional to the old one and not a substitute for it. Experiments with repeated reversal of the same discrimination showed an approach to a random level of attacks. Presumably equal and opposite representations are set up. However, although the total number of attacks declined, the proportion of all attacks that were correct increased. This was probably a result of the plan of the experiment; the food given on each showing of the positive figure served to weight the tendency to attack in favour of that figure. Various interesting phenomena appear with repeated reversal (Mackintosh, 1962; Mackintosh and Mackintosh, 1964 *a* and *b*), but these experiments show no evidence of a specific learning to reverse such as has been found by Harlow and others for birds and mammals. This capacity has not been found in lower vertebrates either (Bitterman, 1965). Reversal is probably one of the special functions that have been added to higher memory systems in the course of evolution.

Errors with Wrong Orientation of the Eyes

A further expectation from our hypothesis would be that alteration of the orientation of the eye or visual field in space should lead to errors of response. This was tested in an ingenious experiment by Wells (1960). After removal of the statocysts from an octopus, when the animal sits on a vertical surface the eye is not held in its normal horizontal position. Wells trained animals to react positively to a horizontal and negatively to a vertical rectangle and then removed the statocysts. When the animal sat on a horizontal surface it continued to perform correctly, but on a vertical surface its responses were erratic or actually reversed.

Conclusion

The hypothesis put forward thus accounts for at least some of the phenomena seen in the learning system of the octopus. No doubt it seems absurdly simplified and "static" to those who are familiar with the subtle learning systems of higher animals. So far as the octopus system is truly simple, it has the advantage of presenting a more easily understandable example, from which we can learn about more complex systems. I have an uneasy feeling, however, that the simplification grossly distorts the picture of the octopus itself. When other aspects of the classifying system are studied it is necessary to postulate additional mechanisms. Sutherland and Mackintosh (1964) postulate that an animal can use one of several classifying systems. It first learns to switch-in whichever system enables it to make a clear discrimination in a new situation. However, the touch memory system can operate when the central nervous system has been so greatly reduced that it is difficult to believe that any elaborate "switching-in" mechanism remains (p. 94).

The code of the nervous system must record many features of the visual world even in an animal as relatively simple as the octopus. This chapter has not tried to deal with all of them, but to show some of the principles upon which they may operate.

CHAPTER THREE

The Requirements of an Exploratory Computer

Signals of Need and Motivation

We have discussed some of the similarities and differences between brains and man-made computers, but we have not yet faced the problems of the design of a computer that explores. Living organisms acquire their own information about the world. More than this, they acquire, over the long process of evolution, their own instructions on how to build and operate an exploratory computer.

By study of the octopus over a number of years some progress has been made toward understanding how its learning system meets the requirements of such a device. Fortunately for the research worker, the octopus brain contains two anatomically distinct and localisable memory stores: one records the results of actions following visual events; the other, the results of actions following the touching of objects with the suckers. Moreover, in each system the actual memory store is accompanied by four lobes of auxiliary equipment. These have been investigated anatomically and experimentally; they seem to be concerned with activities that may be called reading-in to and reading-out from the memory. In particular they serve to send signals of the results of actions to the right addresses in the memory.

These phrases for characterising the functions of the parts must be used with the qualifications that have already been discussed. The nervous memory certainly differs greatly from a magnetic tape. It is by no means certain that we can usefully speak of reading-in to or out from given addresses in it.

Any exploratory learning computer obviously must have a certain bias to take actions. If it does nothing it will learn nothing. We commonly express this by saying that an animal must be motivated. Moreover, it will need detectors that signal when the system lacks essential raw materials, oxygen, food, or water, and these signals must initiate actions that are likely to relieve the need. For example, experiments with implanted electrodes in mammals have shown that feeding behaviour is controlled by paired centres in the hypothalamus. After excision of the lateral centre, a rat starves to death, but after injury of the medial centre he gorges almost literally to the bursting point. The details of the modes of action of such need-centres are only partly understood. Probably they contain the detectors that respond to a lack; this is almost certainly so in the hypothalamic centres that respond to lack of water, and glucoreceptors for sugar are also known.

The presence of such centres in the hypothalamus has been familiar now for some years. It is known that some of the hypothalamic circuits are involved also in recording in the memory. Yet there is little understanding of the principles of the neural mechanisms by which these systems operate. Besides the receptors that indicate the internal state (and hence the "need"), other receptors signal when the appropriate materials arrive (i.e., food or water). These signals must be able to influence the level of motivation and there must be means of adjusting any conflict of requirements. In particular, actions directed to obtaining needed materials must stop if danger threatens, as indicated by signals of pain.

Three Functions of the Signals of the Results of Action

In the octopus the four centres that are connected with each of the two memory systems seem to be concerned, among other things, with signals of taste and of pain (figs. 10 and 11). In these centres, fibres from the lips and mouth interweave with those from the specific receptors (eyes or suckers). Other fibres that probably carry impulses when tissues are damaged (pain) then join in. The two pairs of centres enable these impulses of taste and pain to have their proper effects.

It may be useful to consider what these effects should be to ensure survival of the homeostat. Signals of "reward," indicating to the system the results of its actions, have a series of functions. First, they must operate the appropriate consummatory reactions. When an animal reaches food it must eat; when it touches a very hot object it must withdraw.

Second, the level of exploratory action by the animal must be adjusted. In an unfamiliar situation an animal

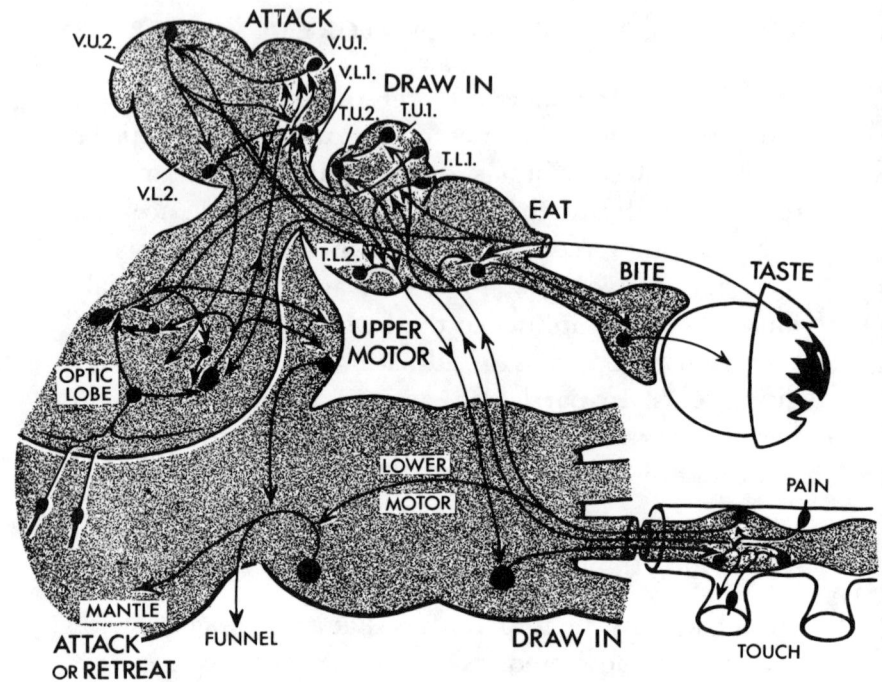

Fig. 10. Diagram of touch and visual learning centres
and their connections in *Octopus*. The suggestion is that
these "higher" centres have developed from "lower" eating centres, and serve to maintain the address of classifying cells between the moment when distance receptors
react and actual contact with the object attacked. Receptors signalling results then deliver signals to the appropriate address. V.L.1, V.L.2, lower visual centres (lateral superior frontal and subvertical). V.U.1, V.U.2, upper
visual centres (median superior frontal and vertical).
T.L.1, T.L.2, lower tactile centres (lateral inferior frontal and posterior buccal). T.U.1, T.U.2, upper tactile
centres (median inferior frontal and subfrontal).

   The pathway from V.U. 2 to T.L. 2 is that by which the
vertical lobe influences touch learning. This is the only
connection between the two systems (except that they
both receive taste and pain fibres). (Modified from Young,
1963*b*)

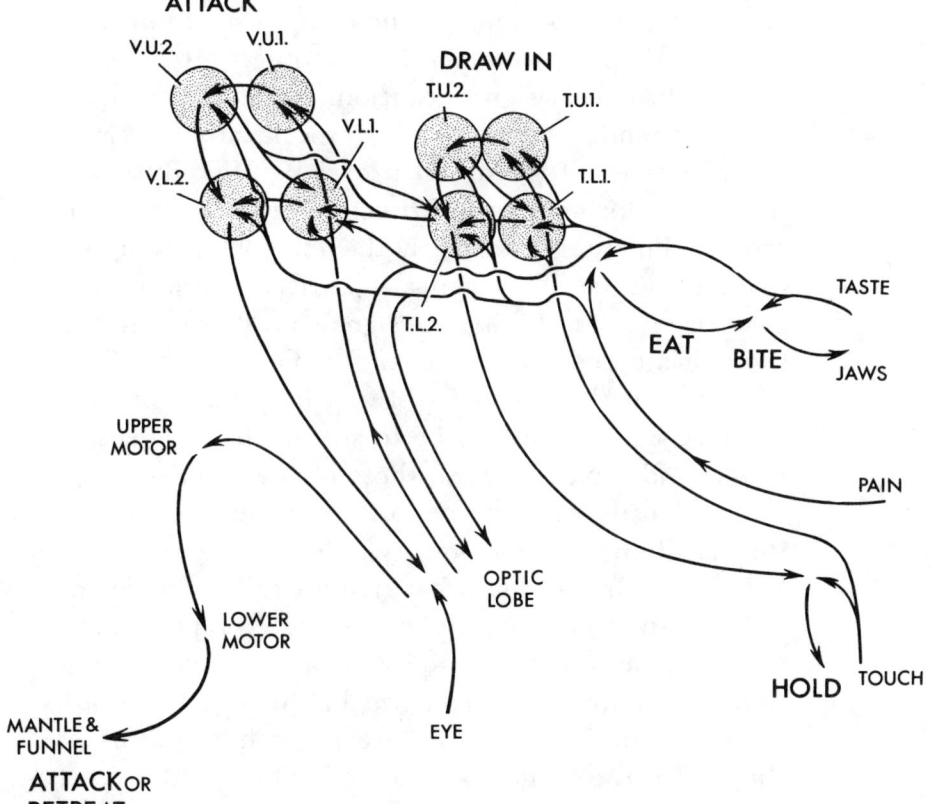

Fig. 11. A more diagrammatic version of figure 10, emphasising similarity of organisation in the touch and visual learning systems. Note mixing of taste and visual information in V.L.1 and V.U.1, and presence of pain fibres entering T.U.2 and V.U.2. (Modified from Young, 1964a)

should proceed cautiously. The octopus does not dash out at full speed to attack a new object. It emerges slowly, with every sign of caution. If the object yields food, the tendency to attack is unspecifically increased and conversely if the object proves painful. But most interesting for us is a third function of these signals of results. They serve to teach the memory specifically that the results of attacking a particular object were good or bad. To do this the signals must reach to the appropriate cells in the memory. One of the chief functions of the two pairs of auxiliary lobes of each memory system seems to be to spread these signals of results and mix them with those of the specific receptors so that they may reach to the appropriate parts of the classifying and memory systems.

It seems obvious that what are here called the signals of the results of action (pleasure, taste or pain) have these various functions to perform. Yet we do not usually find them so described or taught. There are too few situations in which we know how the fibres that carry the signals are routed. One of the chief values of such an analysis is that it directs our attention to the need for investigation of similar pathways and connections in mammals.

The Paired Centres of the Octopus Brain

This analysis has been arrived at, historically, not from first principles but by study of the brain and behaviour of *Octopus*. In this animal two sets of four lobes are connected with the visual and tactile systems respectively. Both sets contain complicated interweaving bundles of fibres. Both sets also include lobes with minute nerve cells—amacrine cells having no axon that leaves the lobe. These centres are so different in appearance from others in the brain that even to look at them suggests that they have special "higher" nervous functions (fig. 12). It was this appearance that led us some years ago to investigate the possibility that they might reveal something about the requirements of neural memory systems. Boycott and I soon found that interruption of the upper visual circuit produces serious defects in the animal's memory for things previously learned and also produces difficulty in further learning. At first we thought that the vertical lobe (second upper visual) was the actual seat of the memory. Then it gradually became clear that animals without that lobe *can* learn, under suitable conditions. Evidently the actual memory record lies elsewhere (in the optic lobe) and the four accessory lobes fulfil special functions, essential for the proper operations of the memory under normal circumstances.

It is not easy to define the functions of these lobes in a few words (perhaps because we have no machines with precisely similar parts). We might list their activities as (1) maintaining the addresses of classifying and memory cells until (2) they deliver to those cells the signals of the results of action (e.g., taste or pain). The paired centres produce these effects by suitable arrangements to mix and circulate signals from specific receptors (vision or touch) with those for taste and pain. They thus acquire as further functions (3) to regulate the level of the tendency to explore and to attack and (4) to transfer representations, especially

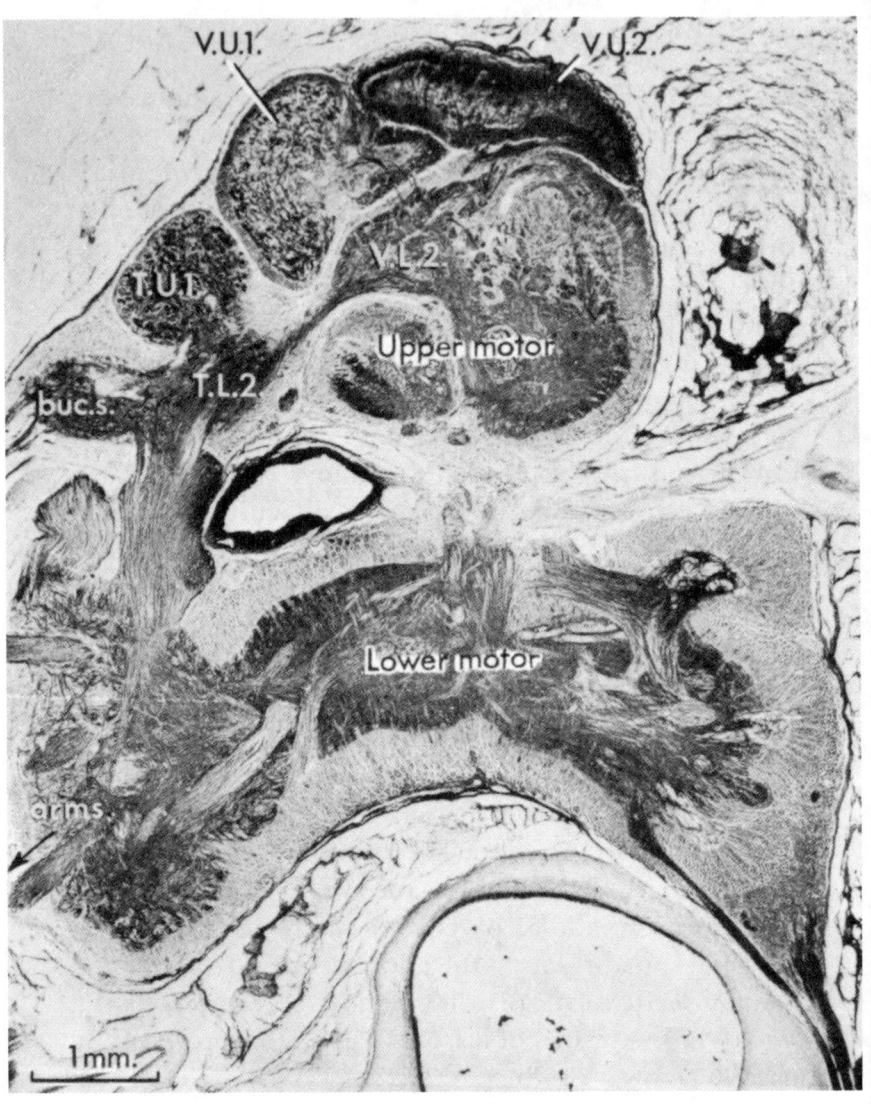

Fig. 12. A vertical longitudinal section cut through whole brain of *Octopus*. Above the gut lie centres for learning and other complex activities. Below it lie centres mediating mainly motor and visceral functions. Optic lobes lie more laterally. buc.s., superior buccal lobe.

from one side of the brain to the other, and to general-
ise them within each receptor field.[1]

This list is only an attempt to summarise the results
of numerous experiments and studies of the connections of the lobes of the octopus brain. It is a measure
of our ignorance of nervous systems that we still cannot easily find words to discuss even these relatively
simple and clearly arranged nerve centres. It is not surprising that we find it so difficult to talk about our own
brains.

To perform their various functions the lobes of both
visual and touch systems are arranged as re-exciting
circuits. They take input from the classifying and
memory systems, combine it with signals of taste and
(or) of pain, and return an output to the memory
centres. Each system has two pairs of centres arranged
in parallel one above the other (fig. 11).

Effects of Lesions to the Lower Visual Circuit

In the visual system we have much experimental evidence about the activities of both the upper and the
lower pairs and are beginning to understand how their
pattern of connections is related to their functions (fig.
13). After interference with the lower visual circuit
the octopus is not blind (fig. 14, operations 6 and 7),
and will still put out an arm to take a crab moving in
the visual field near the animal. The lowest level of
visual function, the seizing of the food, therefore, takes

---

[1] Apparently in *Octopus* there is no generalisation between vision
and touch (see Wells, 1961).

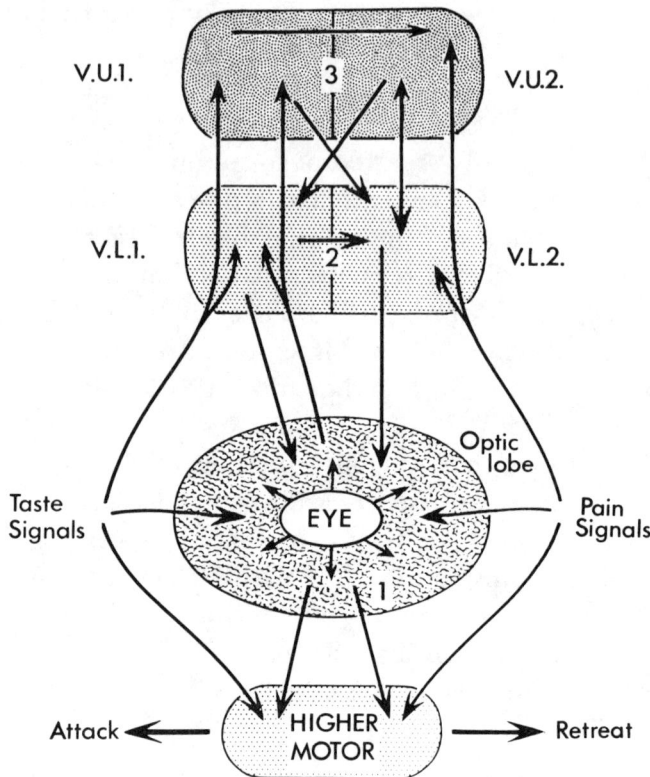

Fig. 13. Diagram of possible functional relationships in visual system. Visual information passes from eye to optic lobe (1). Here it may cause an arm to be put out by activating higher motor centres (basal lobes). Signals of taste and pain reach to the optic lobe, but this system (1) cannot by itself produce a full attack.

Attack requires lower visual circuit (2), which runs through lateral superior frontal and subvertical. Taste and pain fibres also enter these lobes and presumably increase or decrease the probability of attack. Upper visual circuit (3) allows further mixing of visual signals with those of taste, increasing the tendency to attack unless pain intervenes. The pathways shown are mostly well substantiated (though not their functions). Pathway from V.U.1 to V.L.2 is doubtful. (Young, 1964b)

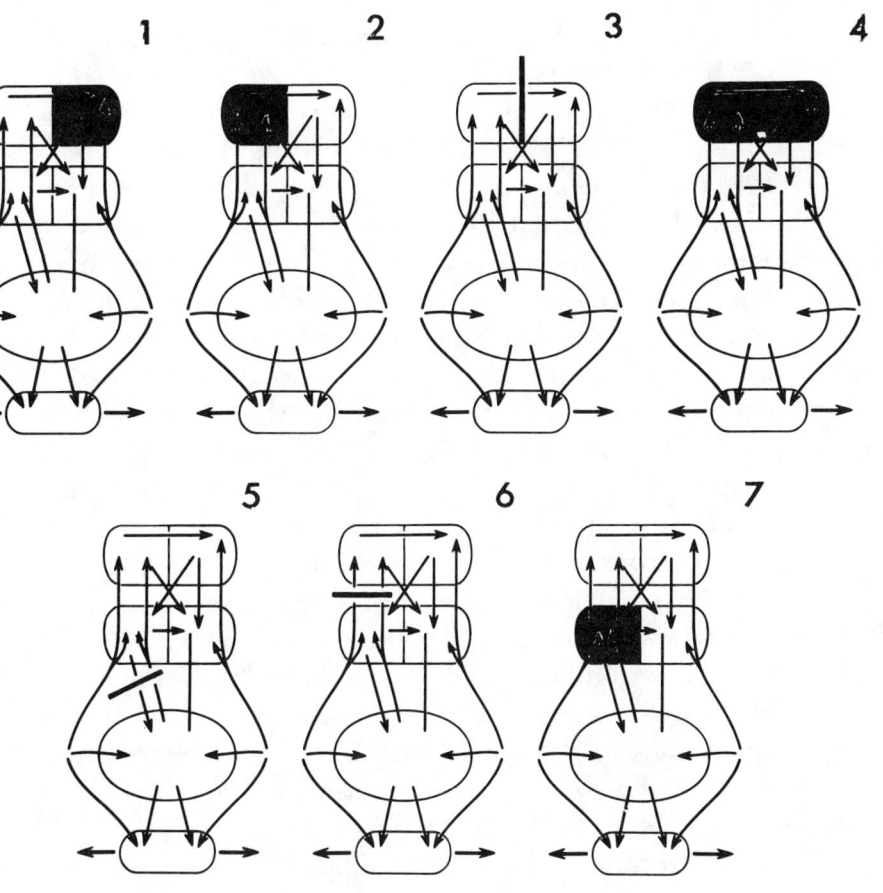

FIG. 14. Diagram showing types of operations performed on *Octopus*. 1. Removal of vertical lobe. 2. Removal of median superior frontal. 3. Cutting of fibre tracts between lateral superior frontal and vertical. 4. Removal of vertical and median superior frontal. 5. Cutting of fibre tracts between optic lobe and median superior frontal. 6. Cutting of fibre tracts between lateral and median superior frontals. 7. Removal of lateral superior frontal. (Young, 1964*b*)

place through the optic lobes alone, in the absence of the paired centres. But such animals never launch out to attack a crab moving at a distance from them. The function of the lower loop thus seems to be to increase the effect of the firing of a few cells of the visual system until it is adequate to produce an attack. This is achieved because each fibre of the input to the visual lower first centre (the lateral superior frontal lobe) runs across the dendritic fields of many cells of the lobe (figs. 14 and 23). There is also an input to the same cells from fibres coming from the region in and around the mouth, presumably taste fibres. Under appropriate circumstances these further increase the tendency to attack.

The axons of the first lower lobe in passing to the visual second lower lobe (subvertical lobe) probably also allow further amplification, since each cell of the first may stimulate many cells of the second. The cells of the lower second visual centre in turn send their axons back to the optic lobes. It is not known clearly what further operations are performed in the second lower lobe. It is the centre of the system in the sense that it receives the output of both the lower and the upper circuits. Its large cells serve to elaborate the "command" that is the final product of the whole system, to be sent back to the optic lobe (see Maldonado, 1963 a, b, c, and d). Fibres presumed to carry pain from all parts of the body also enter the second lower lobe. They may act here to prevent the system from formulating the command to attack if the situation is dangerous.

Because of the central position of the subvertical

lobe in the system, it is impossible to make a separate study of the effects of its removal. Any injury here reduces the tendency of the animal to attack. This must be due mainly to the removal of the effects of the lower pair of centres, because removal of the upper pair produces an animal that in general attacks too much, even in spite of pain (see later).

Connections of the Upper Visual Circuit

The most interesting part of the system is the upper tier of lobes, the median superior frontal and vertical. The mixed bundles of optic and taste fibres proceed through the lateral superior frontal to an astonishing system of interweaving bundles in the median superior frontal (fig. 15). This lobe has a greater proportion of neuropil to its cell layers than any other part of the brain. The incoming fibres run across the dendrite fields of the million small cells of the lobe (fig. 23). This system seems to be designed to allow the setting up of a range of combinations of visual inputs with signals from the chemotactile and taste systems. Any learning system beyond the simplest presumably requires a mechanism to allow for such combinations, and it is striking to see this logical requirement so clearly expressed in the connection pattern, not only here but in almost identical form in the tactile memory system (see later).

The axons of the cells of the first upper lobe pass mainly (probably exclusively) to the second upper lobe (vertical lobe), making as they do so a further elaborate plexus. This plexus ensures that axons of neighbour-

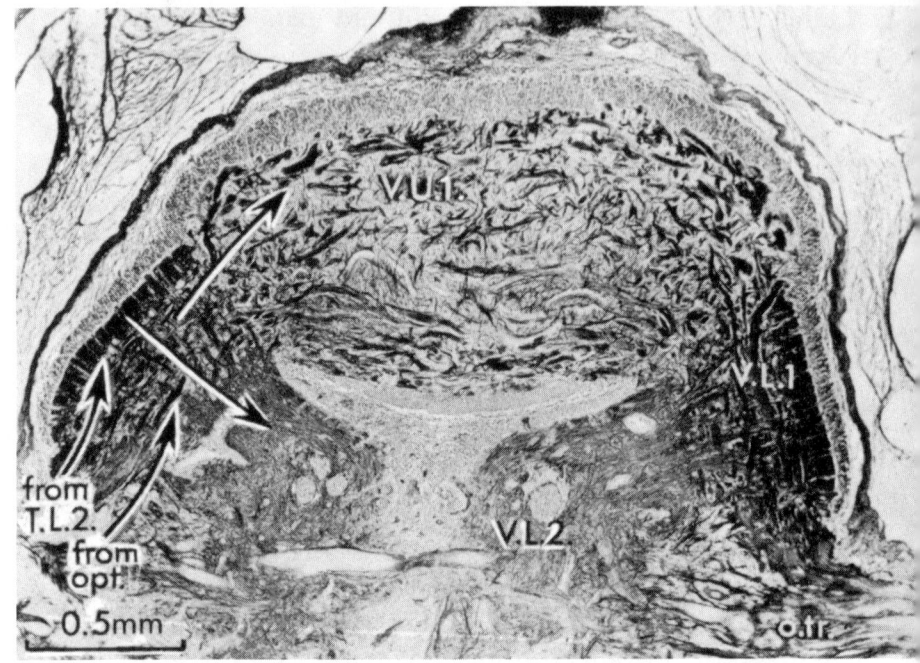

Fig. 15. Transverse section of *Octopus* brain to show lateral and median superior frontal (V.L.1, V.U.1), and subvertical lobes (V.L.2). Note fibre tracts bearing visual information to lateral superior frontal from eye, and fibres from median inferior frontal to lateral superior frontal bearing touch information. In the median superior frontal, the tangled neuropil serves to mix information from these sources. o. tr., optic tract; opt., optic lobe.

ing cells of the first lobe may or may not end near each other in the second lobe and conversely. This is obviously a further system for setting up combinations of activity, perhaps allowing representation of events in the surroundings. A second input to the second upper lobe enters from the subvertical lobe below (fig. 16). It is assumed that these bundles include pain fibres from various parts of the body (see above). The vertical lobe has a very characteristic structure, utterly different from that of the first upper lobe (fig. 23). It contains a vast number of minute amacrine cells (25×10^6) whose fibres do not extend beyond its own neuropil. The output is from a relatively small number of larger cells, with large dendritic fields. They end partly in the second lobe of the lower tier (subvertical), which is thus the output centre for both tiers, transmitting back to the optic lobes. Many other fibres from the second upper lobe pass back to the first lower lobe, providing a feedback, perhaps positive. This may serve to produce the amplification of signals that is necessary to promote or to reduce action.

Failures of Learning after Lesions in the Upper Visual Circuit

Any octopus in which the upper circuit has been interrupted tends to attack more readily than normal, even if the objects that it attacks prove unrewarding or painful (fig. 14, operations 2–5) Boycott and I found that the octopus can be trained by means of shocks not to attack a crab when shown a white square. After the vertical lobe has been removed, however, it immediately

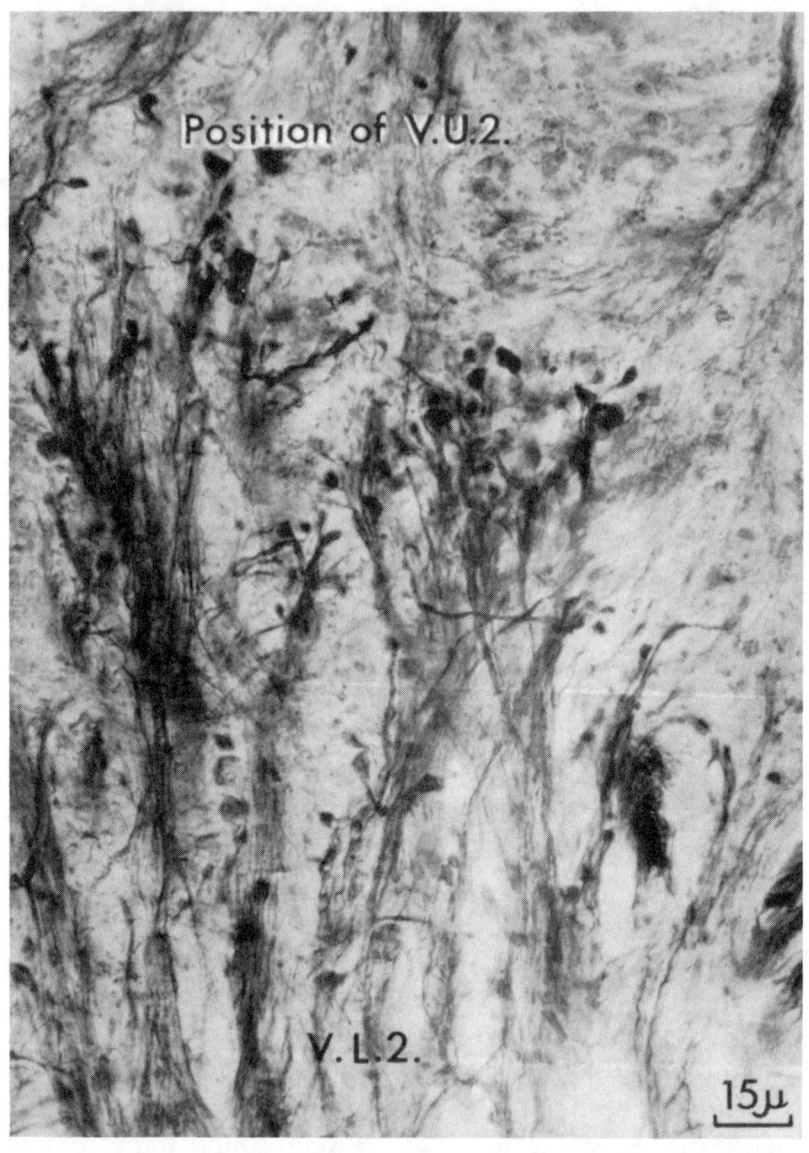

Position of V.U.2.

V.L.2.

15μ

FIG. 16. High-power photograph to show fibres of sub-vertical-vertical tract. The vertical lobe (V.U.2) has been removed, and the ends of nerves leading into it from below are regenerating, as evidenced by swellings at their tips. These fibres are presumed to carry pain signals.

begins to attack again in this situation. If given further shocks for such attacks it will discontinue them, but the memory is effective for only a few minutes. If shocks are given again within that time the record can be maintained, but it lapses if the interval is longer.

The superior frontal to vertical lobe circuit is thus concerned especially in suppressing responses when these lead to painful consequences. The provisional interpretation has been that the actions of the first lobe (median superior frontal) increase the tendency to attack an object that has been seen *unless* pain supervenes, in which case the second (vertical) lobe inhibits the attack tendency. Since the lobes are in series, interference with either may produce similar effects, and there is no doubt that after any operation that interrupts the upper circuit the animal is "uninhibited," in the sense that it attacks more persistently than the normal animal, in spite of pain. However, removal of the median superior frontal and vertical lobes does not produce precisely the same effects. Maldonado (1965) has made a careful comparison of the attacks made at crabs before and after removal of one or other

MEAN TIMES TAKEN TO ATTACK A CRAB $(\frac{1}{100}\text{sec})$[a]

Lobe Removed	Time Before	Days After		
		1—2	3—4	5—6
Median superior frontal	550	2,252	1,667	1,557
Vertical	756	1,057	1,024	1,209

[a] Maldonado, 1965.

of these lobes (see the accompanying table). Animals that attacked crabs at 100 per cent of showings before operation invariably attacked somewhat less thereafter.

Irregularity of response is one symptom of damage to the upper circuit. The reduction in attacks was rather greater if the first lobe was removed than for the second lobe, but great variation occurred in both classes. Much more significant was the fact that the mean time taken for the attacks was much less without the second lobe than without the first.

Maldonado's methods of measurement enabled him to show that this difference was almost wholly in what he calls the "first time delay," that is, the latent period while the animal is still in its home, before the attack is launched. The actual time in transit from home to crab was not greatly different after the two operations.

We can see, therefore, that the upper circuit is concerned in the decision-making process, before the attack begins. The time taken for this process is increased after removing either lobe, but much more so after removing the first lobe than the second. This agrees with the conception that the first lobe is especially concerned with "amplification," or more exactly multiplication, of the signals promoting attack, and the second lobe with inhibiting them.

The structure of the first lobe seems suited to this function. The incoming fibres branch and pass across many of the dendrite fields of the cells of the lobe. Thus impulses in a few incoming fibres may produce many outgoing ones.

The structure of the second (vertical) lobe is so fundamentally different that it must perform some other operation on the circuit. There are strong indications from electron microscopy that the arrangement allows for presynaptic inhibition (figs. 17 and 18). The trunks of the numerous minute amacrine cells of the lobe are packed with synaptic vesicles. They make contact with profiles that also contain vesicles, and have been shown by their degeneration to be the axons of the superior frontal to vertical tract. But the amacrine cells also make conventional synaptic contact with clear profiles in the neuropil, and these are presumed to be the dendritic spines of the large output cells of the lobe.

The endings of the input fibres reaching the lobe from below have not been identified with certainty by means of the electron microscope. However, it is probable that they also make synapse with the amacrine cells. The suggestion is that the incoming fibres from the median superior frontal make excitatory synapses with dendritic spines of the large cells. These pass on the amplified signals *unless* the pain fibres activate the amacrines to release inhibitory transmitter that blocks the incoming impulses. There are possibilities also for postsynaptic inhibition. Indeed, the function of these amacrine cells may be not so much to transmit signals to a distance as to produce an inhibitory clamp (perhaps by depolarisation) upon the system that amplifies the signals to attack.

From the relation between the incoming fibres and the amacrine cells there is good reason to suppose that presynaptic inhibition is involved. Synapses with vesicles on both sides have been found in mammals to be associated with presynaptic inhibition (Wall, 1964; Eccles, 1964). It is very striking that amacrine cells

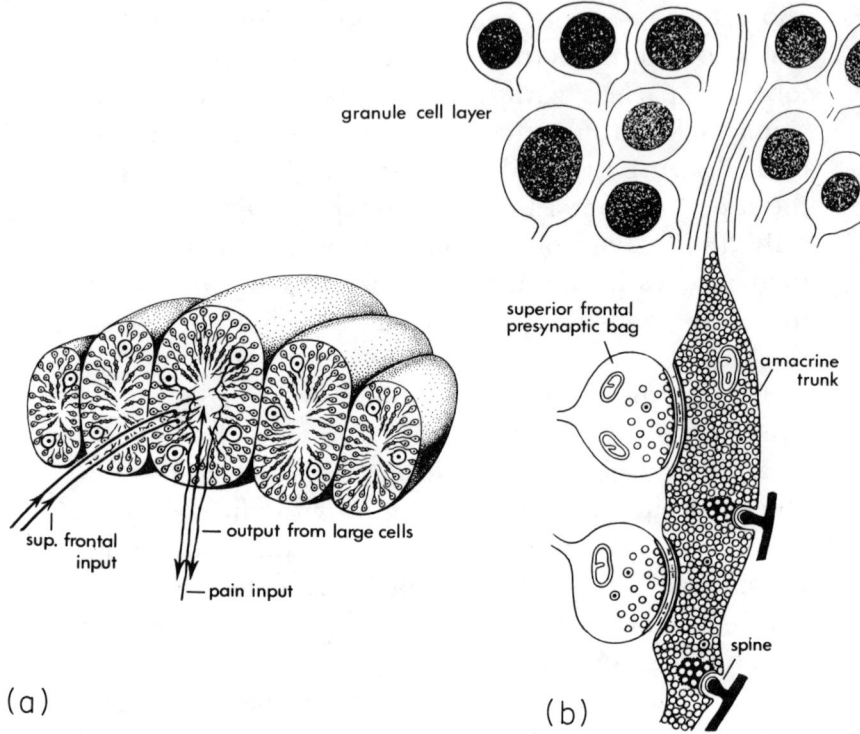

granule cell layer

superior frontal
presynaptic bag

amacrine
trunk

sup. frontal
input

— output from large cells

— pain input

spine

(a)

(b)

FIG. 17. Diagrams of vertical lobe of *Octopus*. *a*, arrangement of cells and fibres; note input of axons from median superior frontal lobe. *b*, connections in vertical lobe as revealed by electron microscopy. Median superior frontal fibres terminate in typical presynaptic bags, containing vesicles of presumed transmitter substance, which abut against processes of amacrine cells of vertical lobe. These processes are packed with transmitter vesicles, and would appear to pass on stimulation to clear spinous processes of unknown origin, perhaps dendrites of the large output cells. Synapses of the pain fibres not shown. (Gray and Young, 1964)

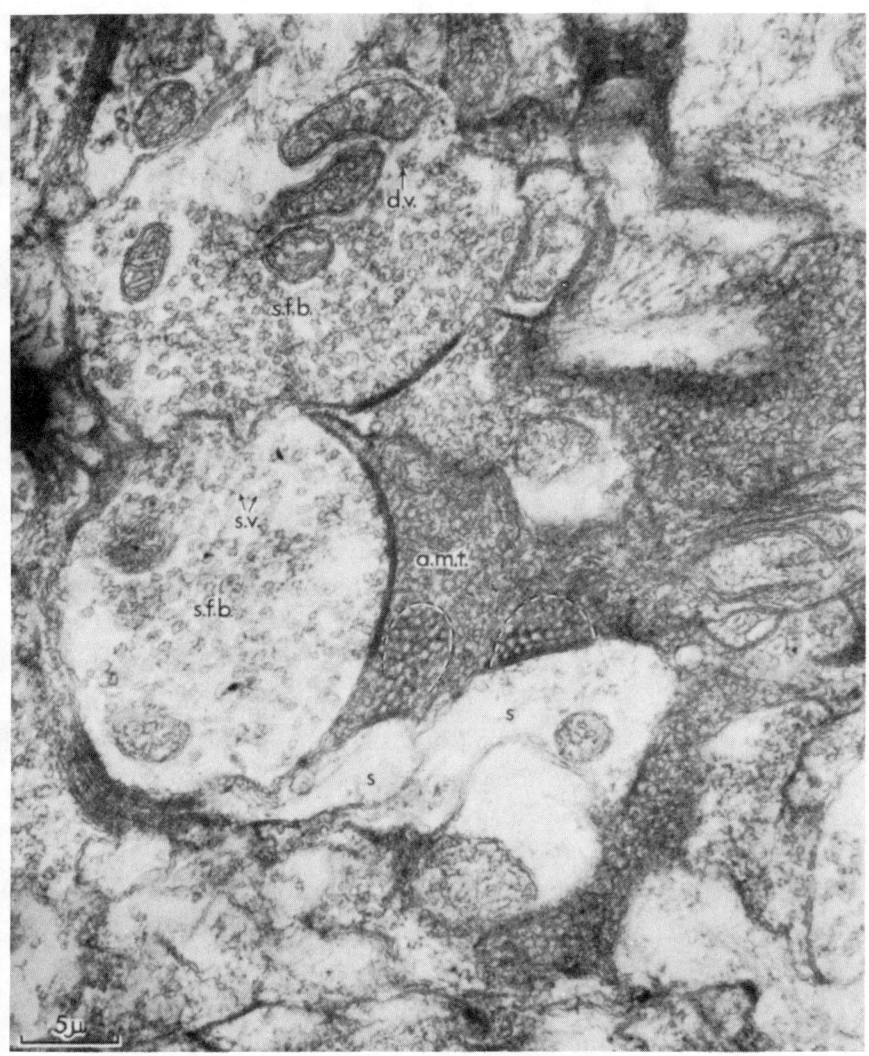

Fig. 18. Electron micrograph of the vertical lobe, showing superior frontal fibres, s.f.b., filled with vesicles, making contact with an amacrine cell; a.m.t. This is also
filled with vesicles, and is in turn in contact with spines,
s., which have no vesicles. d.v., dense-centred vesicle; s.v.,
synaptic vesicle. (Gray and Young, 1964)

and synapses with vesicles on both sides are totally absent from the median superior frontal lobe.

Although we do not fully understand the workings of the vertical lobe system, the experiments begin to show various clues to its place in the learning mechanism. Animals from which the vertical lobe is removed show at first no capacity to learn to attack one figure that yields food (say a horizontal rectangle), while not attacking another that gives a shock (say a vertical rectangle), *if these are shown successively* (fig. 19). Not uncommonly they continue to attack each figure at every presentation. This experiment does not show that the actual memory record lies in the vertical lobe system. If the animals are then tested by showing figures alone, without giving either rewards or shocks, they attack the "positive" figure more often than the "negative," although they had previously shown no sign of learning. The responses remain erratic, but are more often right than wrong, showing that something had been learned.

This result may be interpreted as indicating that a record can be written in the optic lobes, more or less correctly, even when they act by themselves, but that without the vertical lobes the record is not properly used or "read-out." When the animal takes food, the tendency to attack is unduly raised, and the record in the memory that prevents attack at the negative figure is not used. An attack occurs in spite of the record in the memory.

This is confirmed by training operated animals in a simultaneous discrimination situation. They now perform reasonably well, though less accurately than nor-

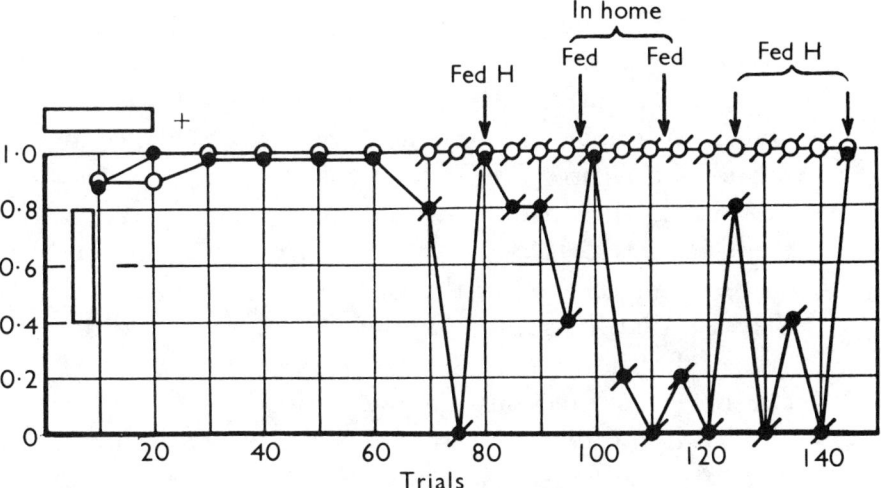

Fɪɢ. 19. Plot of responses of an octopus with 85% of the vertical lobe removed. Trained to attack a horizontal but to avoid a vertical rectangle (solid circles) it seemed to learn nothing in 60 trials, attacking nearly every time. In a series of tests without rewards (all barred circles) performance was correct, but again deteriorated when food was given (at the points shown with arrows). This happened whether the food was given in the home (Fed H) or with the horizontal rectangle. (After Young, 1958)

mal control animals (Muntz, Sutherland, and Young, 1962). In this situation the system must choose one of the two alternatives, whatever the attack level may be, and the information in the memory tips the balance in favour of the correct response.

Animals that had been trained before operation seem at first to have lost all capacity for correct response after removal of the vertical lobes (fig. 20). If they are then re-trained, however, they recover a degree of discrimination. This again shows that a record can be established outside the vertical lobe system. However, the performance was much more accurate when trials were given at intervals of five minutes than at hourly intervals. Much re-learning took place within each session (when trials were given at five-minute intervals) and was then forgotten before the next set of trials began six to twelve hours later. This again can be interpreted by supposing that the vertical lobe system is somehow concerned with maintaining the representation for a sufficient period for it to be "printed" in the more permanent memory.

The Upper Visual Circuit and Transfer of Representations

The demonstration that the actual record is not in the vertical lobe system makes the analysis of the functions of the vertical lobe all the more revealing. One striking result of interrupting its circuit is to prevent transfer to the other side of the body of a representation that is set up by training with only one eye. It was shown by Muntz (1961) that the octopus is particularly suitable

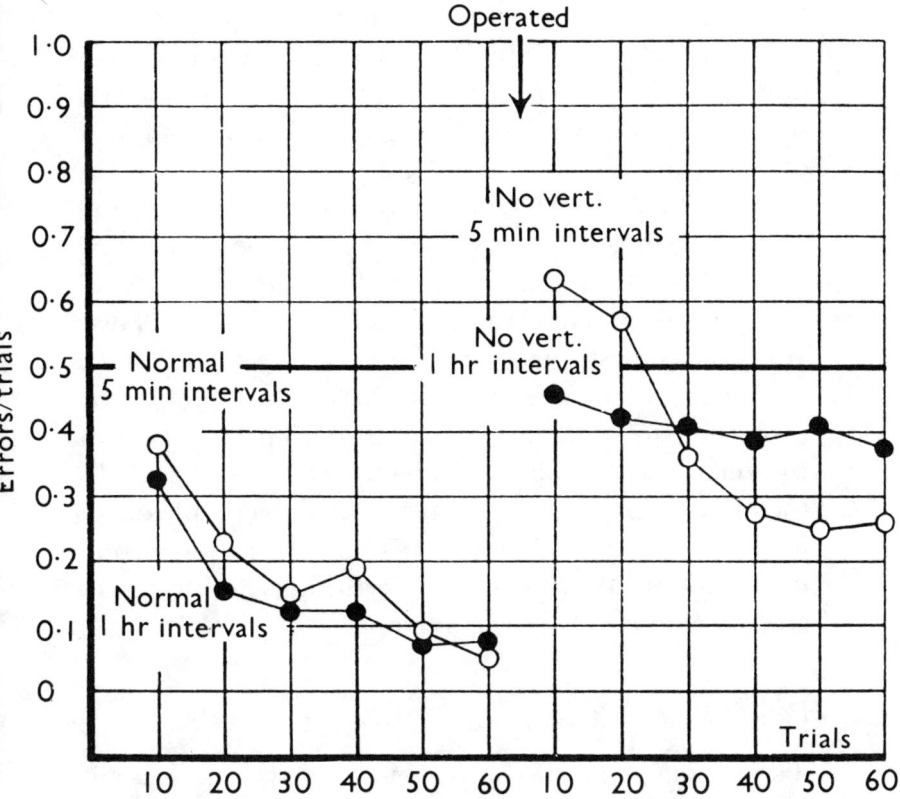

Fig. 20. Plot of the responses of 10 octopuses given trials at 5-minute intervals, and 10 at 60-minute intervals. Before and after removal of the vertical lobe (vert.). Food was given for attack at a horizontal rectangle (open circles), shock for attack at a vertical one (solid circles). Before operation the 5-minute group was slightly the more accurate. After operation it was initially less accurate, but finally more accurate than the 60-minute group. Thus the vertical lobe may serve to hold short-term memory before storage in the optic lobe. (After Young, 1960b)

for such experiments. The input can be given to one eye only and the optic lobe of that side then removed. The animal will perform correctly with the other eye, but only if the vertical lobe circuit had been intact during training. This is all the more interesting because the large optic commissure directly connecting the two optic lobes is left intact by the operation. The hypothesis is that the fibres of this commissure serve to connect similar classifying cells on the two sides. When cells classifying for horizontal are activated on one side, similar ones are made active on the other by the actions of the optic commissure. The function of the vertical lobe would then be to deliver to these cells the appropriate signals of taste or pain. The plexus of fibres of the tract that connects the first and second upper lobes allows many opportunities for fibres to cross from one side to the other.

Paired Centres in Sepia

The arrangement of the vertical lobe system, as a circuit re-exciting the optic lobes, suggests that it acts as a positive feedback, increasing the effect of the signals of taste on the memory cells. The internal feedback within the vertical lobe system may well further increase the effect. The significance of self re-exciting systems has been much debated. Many years ago, when a similar circuit was found in the vertical lobe system of *Sepia,* reverberation was suggested as the basis of the memory record (Young, 1938). The vertical lobe system of *Sepia* is simpler than that of *Octopus,* for it has no median superior frontal lobe. Fibres from a lobe with structure somewhat similar to that of the lateral superior frontal of *Octopus* proceed directly to the vertical lobe (fig. 21). From the latter, fibres run partly to the subvertical and thence to the optic lobe, and partly as a feedback to the superior frontal.

Little is known about learning in *Sepia,* but it was shown that the animals are capable of pursuing their prey (a prawn) when it disappears behind a rock (Sanders and Young, 1940). This simple form of memory would be valuable for a cuttlefish. After removal of the vertical lobe the animals were unable to hunt in this way. When a prawn disappeared from sight the cuttlefish without vertical lobe abandoned the search. The suggestion made at the time was that in a normal *Sepia* reverberation maintains what would now be called a "representation" of the prawn (Young, 1938). It is curious that this suggestion was made when, so far as I can remember, I had never heard about self re-exciting circuits in electrical engineering. I had of course read about them in the experiments and discussions of Lorente de Nó (1936) in relation to the control of eye movements.

Paired Centres and Addressing in the Memory

No one now considers that the permanent record in the brain is a continuous circulating memory, but probably even in mammals circulation plays an important part in maintaining the representation until it is printed. The significance of self re-excitation may be that it bridges the time gap, inevitable when any distance receptor is stimulated, between activation of

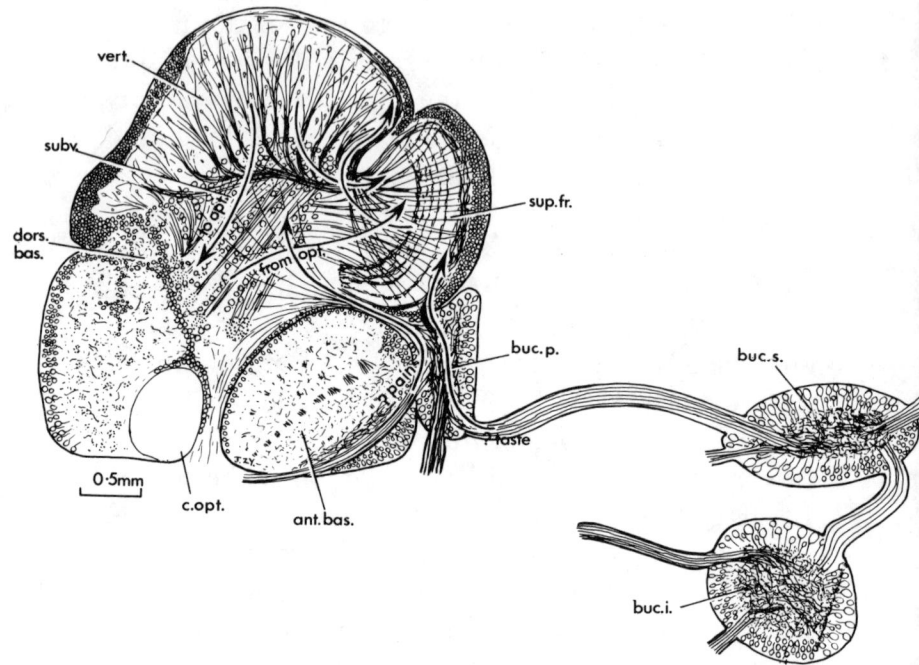

FIG. 21. Drawing of a vertical longitudinal section through the brain of *Sepia*, a decapod. Note that the visual learning system—superior frontal (sup. fr.), vertical (vert.), subvertical (subv.)—is as in *Octopus* but simpler. There is a simpler touch system since decapods rely less on touch than do octopods. The superior buccal is far forward, and there is no inferior frontal or subfrontal. ant. bas., anterior basal lobe; dors. bas., dorsal basal lobe; buc.s., superior buccal lobe; buc.i., inferior buccal lobe; buc.p., posterior buccal lobe; c.opt., optic commissure. (Young, 1963*b*)

the classifying cells and arrival of the signals indicating the result of the action taken. One function of the vertical lobe circuit is probably to maintain the addresses of the classifying cells that have been stimulated and then to deliver to them the appropriate signals when they arrive. In physiological terms this would consist in maintaining the relevant cells at a lowered threshold, perhaps by depolarisation.

A function of this sort is indicated by the fact that the octopus without a vertical lobe has especial difficulty in learning not to attack a figure that is unrewarding or painful (Boycott and Young, 1950). Under some circumstances the operated animal can do so only if trials are repeated at very short intervals. However, it is surprising that an octopus without a vertical lobe is still able to make delayed responses. If a crab is placed under one of two cups which the octopus is looking at from behind glass, when released it will choose the right one up to a minute later. This capacity is not lost after removal of the vertical lobe (Dilly, 1963).

Removal of the vertical lobe has shown that it is not the seat of the visual memory record, but is concerned with the establishment and use of that record, as we may say with reading-in and reading-out. How justifiable it is to use these terms remains to be seen. The nervous memory, it may be said, is not a detailed addressed record. But in conventional experiments on conditioning, maze learning, or discrimination we do not usually examine the system with the aims of discovering whether there are records of individual occasions of learning. We are so used to the concept of repeated "trials" as a part of the learning procedure that we forget that characteristic events must happen at each trial. This change at a single occasion of learning, rather than the study of results of repeated trials, should be the goal of physiological enquiry.

We know that the human brain is able to store a record of individual occasions and that this record lasts for many years. In man there is much to indicate that the first time of presentation of a situation is recorded with especial accuracy. Experiments with animals are seldom conducted with a view to discovering whether this is so for them also. To be useful in the wild state the memory must be able to establish records as a result of a relatively small number of occasions. Man and higher animals undergo a long period of learning to learn, during which the "model" is built up in the brain. Once a general representation of the world around is established, a record of the detailed results of fresh experiments can be added very rapidly. Perhaps one of the ways in which a simple memory like that of the octopus differs from our own is that it does not have to learn to learn. Heredity endows the octopus with the power to form quickly associations between relatively few features detected in the environment and the food value or pain that accompanies them. Incidentally, it is of great importance that not everything should be recorded in the memory, and that some items should be held for a short time and then erased. Indeed, "attention" ensures that only a part of the sensory input is filtered through for possible storage in the memory.

*Addressing in the Memory and the Stream of
Consciousness*

The mechanism for reading-in to and reading-out from
the memory throws light on the problem of the basis
of individuality, including that of man. Although the
brain is continuously bombarded with impulses from
different receptors and along many channels, yet an
animal or man pursues one more or less consistent line
of action. Again, each human being follows one stream
of consciousness. We "consult the memory" about one
question at a time.

These are striking facts in spite of their familiarity,
and they suggest that there must be a mechanism that
ensures unity of action, and in particular performs an
operation that could properly be called "consulting
the memory." There is indeed some evidence that the
appropriate mechanism is included in the reticular
system, which lies at the centre of the gray matter
throughout the brain and spinal cord. This system includes neurons that are activated from an exceptionally wide range of afferent sources (Jasper *et al.*,
1958). Efferent neurons from the system reach to many
parts of the brain, including the thalamus and cortex.
Stimulation of it influences the state of sleeping and
produces "arousal responses" in the cortex.

Penfield has long held, as a result of his studies by
stimulation of the human brain, that some "cen-
trencephalic system" must exist at the centre of the
human personality (see Penfield and Roberts, 1959).
It is not possible at present to be very specific, al-

though the problem is crucial for discussion of the nature of the memory system, at least in higher animals.

Systems for selective reading-in and reading-out are likely to be present as important and distinct mechanisms. As we have seen, they appear to be prominent in the octopus. We already possess a considerable amount of information about such systems in mammals. It is no accident that the centres in the hypothalamus that are concerned with establishing the level of need, as in food consumption, are also involved in consummatory acts such as feeding or defence. To initiate such actions is the primary function of the signals of results, taste and pain.

The same regions are involved also in circuits that are essential for recording in the memory. In man, defects of memory follow lesions in the hippocampus (if bilateral) or the mammillary bodies (e.g., Korsakoff's disease). The power affected is that of recording recent events; records already established are not impaired. In some respects the parallel with the vertical lobe system is striking; it suggests that the basal forebrain circuits are concerned with reading-in to the memory and, specifically, with maintaining the "addresses" of the classifying cells, presumably in the neocortex, and sending to them the signals of results. This hypothesis suggests that it would be worth while to look again at the pathways between the limbic system and the neocortex, which would be concerned with such addressing. These structures all form part of a complex system of circuits in which the hippocampus sends impulses down through the fornix to the mammillary bodies. From here fibres pass to the anterior nucleus of the thalamus and thence up again to the cingulate gyrus and so perhaps to other parts of the cortex and back to the hippocampus.

It has long been known that the limbic system somehow constitutes a "circuit of emotion" (Papez). We now begin to see how the involvement in "emotion" may be due to the fact that the system includes not only circuits of "needs" but also of "rewards." Rewards have the function of exciting not only consummation but also memory. Injuries in the hypothalamus or limbic system may thus disturb the whole or parts of the motivational and consummatory system as well as the memory records that go with them. We are only beginning the search for a clear language to speak and write about these centres, which so nearly affect our personality and well-being. It is curious that little attention has been given in the past to the question how nerve impulses in fibres signalling taste or pain can reach to all parts of the memory system of a mammal. They must somehow do so if they are to teach it. We have lacked a model that would suggest what questions may be asked about the connections of the memory. The octopus system, by its relative simplicity, reveals certain features that we may look for in higher nervous systems.

The Chemotactile Learning System of Octopus

Perhaps the strongest confirmation that our analysis of the functions of these circuits is on the right track is that the whole set of lobes is repeated in the part of

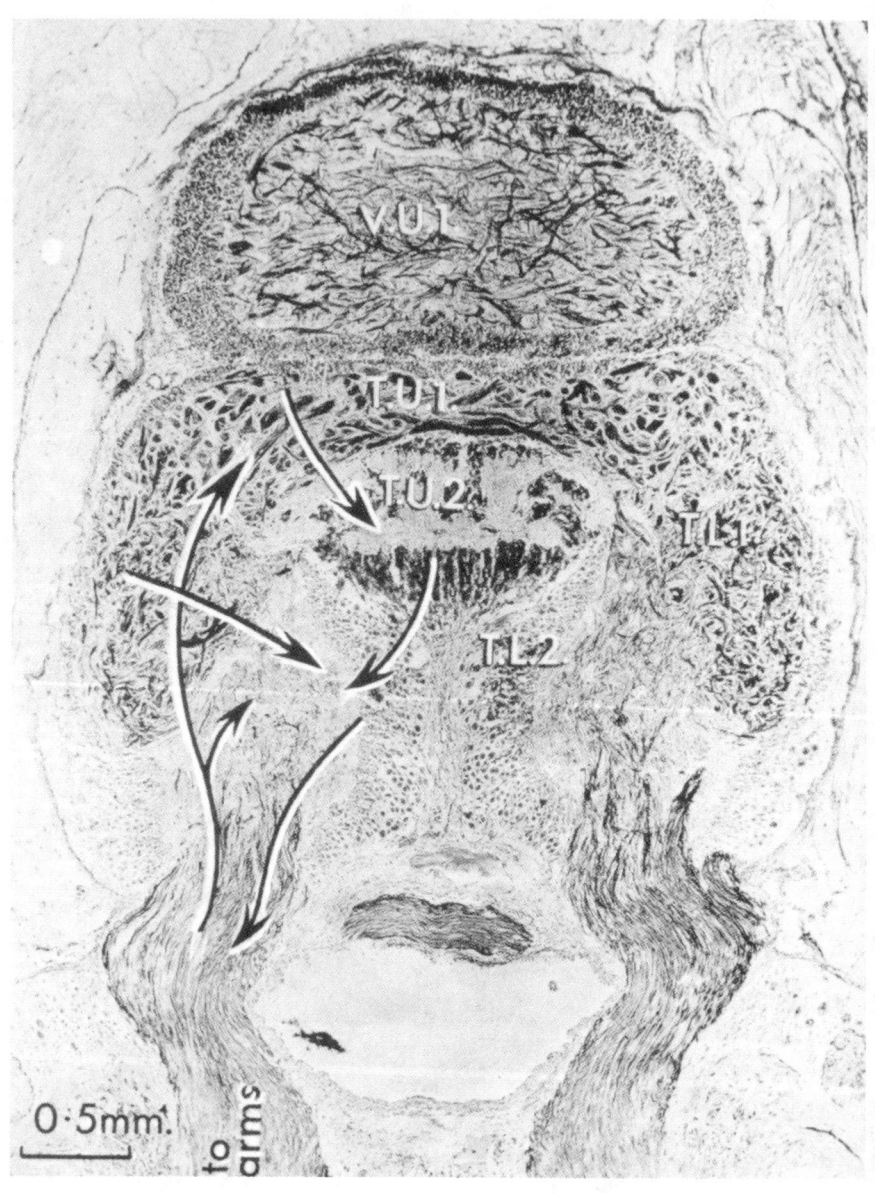

Fig. 22. Transverse section of octopus brain to show centres associated with touch learning. (Abbreviations as in fig. 10)

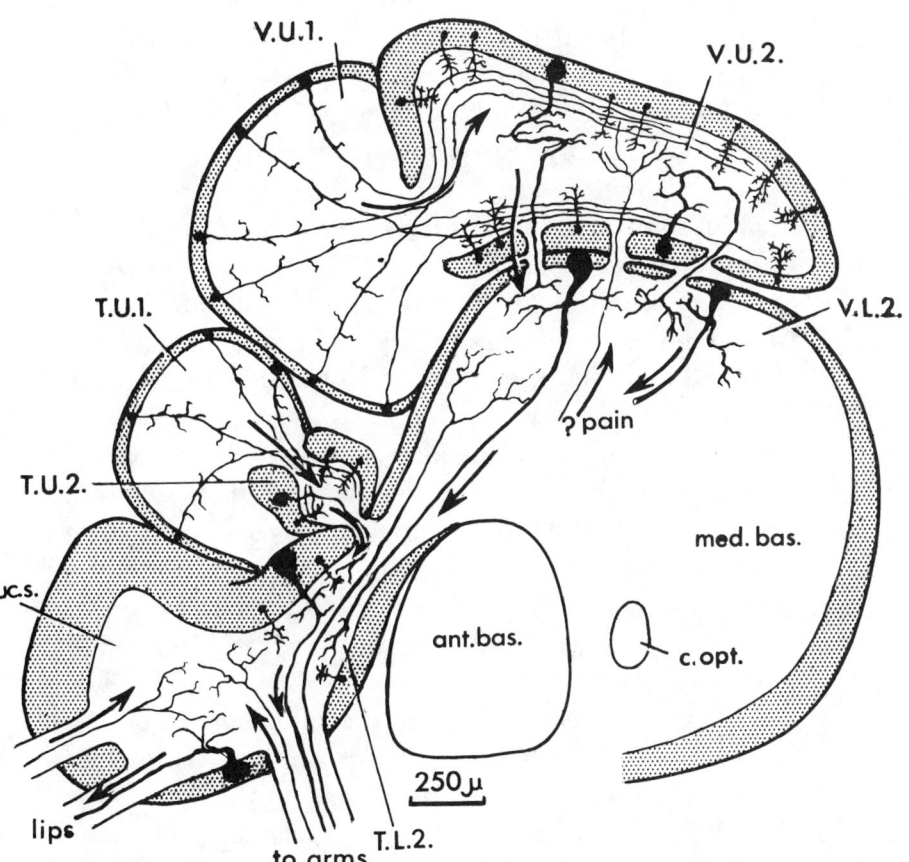

FIG. 23. Diagram of selected cells from various learning centres of octopus brain as revealed by Golgi stain.
Compare with figs. 10 and 11. med. bas., median basal
lobe. (Other abbreviations as in figs. 10 and 21) (Young,
1963*b*)

the octopus brain that is concerned with learning to discriminate between objects by touch (figs. 22 and 23). Mr. and Mrs. Wells have established (1957) that the animal readily learns to take a rough object but rejects a smooth one. Incidentally, the octopus was unable to distinguish objects by shape alone (i.e., square from cube) or by weight. As the Wellses point out, the amount of positional information coming from a flexible arm that lacks joints probably makes it intolerably difficult to compute its spatial distribution.

The part of the brain that is concerned with touch has four lobes closely similar to those of the visual system, though somewhat less sharply distinct from each other. There is no centre exactly corresponding to the optic lobe, but Wells showed that no learning is possible if the tactile lower second lobe (posterior buccal) is removed. This region of large and small cells apparently functions as the memory store itself. The system is less specialised than the visual one, and the posterior buccal lobe corresponds both to the second lower visual centre (subvertical) and to the optic lobe. This is perhaps a result of the fact that the touch memory is a relatively recent acquisition; hence no distinct tactile lobe comparable to the optic lobe has yet been evolved.

After interference with the upper circuit of the tactile system, simple discriminations can still be made. As in the visual system, these lobes are not the seat of the memory, but are needed for its proper use in more difficult discriminations. Moreover, they are concerned in transfer; after their removal a discrimination that had been learned by teaching only one arm or one side of the body is not performed by the others. Removal of these lobes does not in any way impair visual learning, and removal of the optic lobes does not influence the tactile memory. This is very striking when it is remembered that the optic lobes together weigh more than twice as much as all the rest of the brain. They contain 120,000,000 cells against 40,000,000 in the central ganglia. The entire section of the central system that pertains to touch learning contains 6,400,000 cells; 5,000,000 of these are the minute amacrine cells of the subfrontal lobes (Young, 1963 a). Of course the arms contain many cells concerned with touch, but the arm centres by themselves are incapable of learning.

In the octopus, then, visual and tactile memory functions are sharply localised. Yet the two systems are not wholly independent. Wells and Wells (1957) showed that touch learning is unduly slow after removal of the vertical lobe. This will no doubt prove to be another valuable clue to the vertical lobe functions.

We can be encouraged in our search for the principles of recording in the memory by finding these two sets of pairs of centres in the visual and tactile learning systems. Their plans of connection are exceptionally clear and precise. We do not yet fully understand them, even after years of work, but the basic design is beginning to appear. However wrong our interpretations may be in detail, they cannot be wholly so. The sets of pairs of centres are there. They have been proved to play a part in the learning of the octopus. They may provide hints as to the way to study some features of learning in higher animals.

CHAPTER FOUR

The Nature of the Memory Record and the Origin of Learning

Some Essential Features of Neural Memory Systems

A hypothesis that is likely to lead us toward discovery of the changes that occur in a neural memory is that learning consists in the limitation of choice between alternatives. The setting up of a representation in the memory of the nervous system is like the printing of a book in that it involves selecting appropriate items from a pre-established alphabet. We have evidence that such a repertoire exists. Each animal species has limited capacities to react to features of the external environment. Presumably it is similarly limited in the ability to make records in its memory. Brains are not general-purpose computers but specialised analogues. We must qualify this statement, because in the not unimportant case of our own brains we achieve a high degree of generality. In the evolution of the memory mechanisms of primates there has been a gradual release from dependence on the classifying systems built in by heredity. It is worth while to consider how this freedom has been achieved. It has apparently reached the point that the human brain at birth is almost a blank sheet ready to memorise anything. To do this is obviously the goal of the perfect learning homeostat, able to adapt to any environment. If we consider what a feat it would be to succeed in doing this we may be reminded that even our apparently powerful human brain is probably more specialised and limited than we realise. This may also remind us of the urgent need for further study of the human coding and classifying system and of its development, so that we may learn how to train it more efficiently. Until we know something of the principles of the operation of the memory, educational theory can only proceed empirically, with no real scientific basis.

It may be, however, that it is desirable to study first the methods of recording in simpler memory systems than our own. The fact that we are only just beginning to be able to recognise the nature of the problem shows the urgent need for a strategy that may proceed logically from well-understood simpler systems toward our own complicated one.

What essential features would be expected in a neural memory system? It is of little use to study chemical or electrical changes in the brain, or to look for synaptic alterations, unless we first decide what sort of system we are looking for and hence where the changes are likely to be. The need for a logical strategy is imposed on us by the fact that the brain is a multichannel system, with numerous parts of very small size. There are probably at least 10,000 synaptic points on one large cortical neuron (perhaps many more). How many of these would be altered when an animal has learned? Would they all change at once? Would some have been changed by previous learning? Worse still, there must be thousands of synaptic vesicles in a single presynaptic terminal. If learning consists in the production of a flood of inhibitory or excitatory transmitter, what changes, if any, should we expect to see in the vesicles? How many would be changed? The electron microscope is perhaps the one instrument with the resolution in space that is required to see changes, but we must know where to look. So far, we have no evidence on whether the changes are presynaptic (e.g., in the vesicles) or whether they occur in the transmitting or receiving properties of the synaptic membranes.

Some Hypotheses on the Mechanism of Learning

The microelectrode has about 1,000 times less resolution in space than the electron microscope, but its resolution in time is millions of times greater. It has already provided some interesting evidences of changes during learning, which it is not possible to summarise here (see Jasper and Smirnov, 1960). There is evidence of persistence of the effects of volleys of stimuli (post-tetanic potentiation or depression). When an animal is subjected to rhythmical stimuli the appropriate rhythm may appear in the brain, at least in some stages of learning, especially in the hippocampus (Adey *et al.*, 1960; Jasper *et al.*, 1958). Characteristic patterns of electrical activity can be transmitted across the brain to mirror foci and can be made to endure there (Morrell, 1960, 1961). Such results provide valuable clues, but they do not show how the changes serve the function of writing a particular record in the memory.

It is difficult to evaluate the work of Hydén (1960), who identifies the record as written by changes in the base ratios of ribosenucleotides in the nerve cells. The technique used, which makes possible the study of single cells, at least approaches the spatial resolution that is needed. To identify changes in base ratios in single cells is indeed a feat. The results suggest that some modification of the RNA is included in the learning changes. As Hydén has emphasised, these nucleotides are so abundant in nerve cells that it would be strange if they were not involved in the memory. It is not yet possible to see exactly how the changes that Hydén reports are connected with the actions that were learned, for example, by a rat balancing upon a wire. It would not be easy to specify exactly what alterations in motor pattern are concerned. Most serious of all, it is difficult to believe that the coding system includes the volleys of impulses of specifically timed frequency that Hydén's theory seems to require, or that these frequencies would be in the right range to control the synthesis of specific RNA's.

However, there seems to be evidence that changes in RNA base ratios do occur during learning, and this is to be expected. It does not necessarily follow that the changes in the RNA specifically embody the particular item to be recorded. A characteristic feature of brains as multichannel systems is that they achieve specificity by allowing particular channels for each item in the alphabet, rather than by passing coded signals along each channel. Similarly for the memory, our hypothesis here will be that each item is written in the memory by changing the state of a particular set of cells. The capacity for such change is almost certainly dependent upon the cell nucleotides and they themselves may well alter with the change. But the item recorded is not a function of the particular nucleotide change; it is a feature that the cell was pre-set to record. In this pre-setting, achieved during embryological development, the cell nucleotides provide the instructions by which a memory capable of recording certain items is built.

Learning by Closing Unneeded Channels

The thesis here advanced is that it may prove possible to make further progress by considering situations in which the record made in the memory during learning is the result of a choice between two specific alternatives. Most behaviour is compounded of a series of choices. For our purposes it is convenient to study situations in which the animal clearly does one of two things according to the record in its memory. In the octopus we have two such situations: the attack or retreat when some object moves in the visual field, and the taking or rejecting of an object by the arms. We know something of the cells and pathways that are involved and we can draw up a scheme for the process of recording in the memories. Moreover, we can form some idea how these memory systems have arisen from a state in which the brain was not capable of learning.

If the classifying cells of the visual system have been correctly identified we may suppose that they have outputs that can lead to either attack or retreat. The learning change consists, as suggested in the second chapter, in closing one of these channels (fig. 8). This may be brought about through collaterals of the cells, here labelled "memory cells" (because they provide the alternatives for choice). These collaterals may activate the small cells, of which there are many in the cell islands of the optic lobes, causing them to block the alternative pathway. There is little evidence, unfortunately, about the details of the anatomy or connections of the cells at the centre of the optic lobes—a vast tangle of fibres which has not been adequately described with the light microscope, let alone with the electron microscope. Small cells accompanying large are commonly found in this region, as in the parts of the brains that are thought to be responsible for learning in vertebrates and arthropods. They are found again in the touch learning centres of an octopus. It has been suggested for many years that some of the small cells in the spinal cord have the function of producing an inhibitory transmitter in a pathway (see Wall, 1964; Eccles, 1964). The present suggestion is that in centres that learn this process has been extended. These small cells have become specialised, with the result that upon receipt of appropriate signals they manufacture or release enough inhibitor to block the alternative path for a long time, perhaps permanently. There are many ways in which this could be achieved. In the vertical lobe, numerous small cells make serial synapses, at which there are vesicles on both sides of the membrane. These may well be sites of presynaptic inhibition. It is possible that the small cells of the optic lobes are similar and that they can produce a flood of inhibitor around the presynaptic junctions. Perhaps there is a suitably triggered enzyme system, itself held inhibited, to be released at the appropriate signal. The analogy of the mechanisms of genetic control is obvious and may suggest experimental approaches. The connection with the RNA metabolism may be found in the special mechanisms of synthesis of inhibitor that are needed.

It is not profitable to speculate further, but the hypothesis can in principle be tested at the chemical level, though little is yet known of synaptic transmitters in Cephalopods (see Welsh, 1961). Perhaps the touch learning system is even more suitable for study than the visual one. Wells showed originally, and he and I have recently confirmed, that learning to take a rough object and to reject a smooth one can take place with relatively few large cells, surrounded by a few tens of thousands of minute ones (figs. 24 and 25). Moreover, in animals functionally bisected we have been able to teach the two sides in opposite directions. There is here a wonderful material that has perhaps as much simplicity as can be expected in a learning system. When all the higher parts of the brain have been removed, the octopus lies as a postureless preparation, yet it is able, as soon as it touches an object, to draw it in or push it away. It is worth directing microelectrodes, electron microscopes, and microspec-

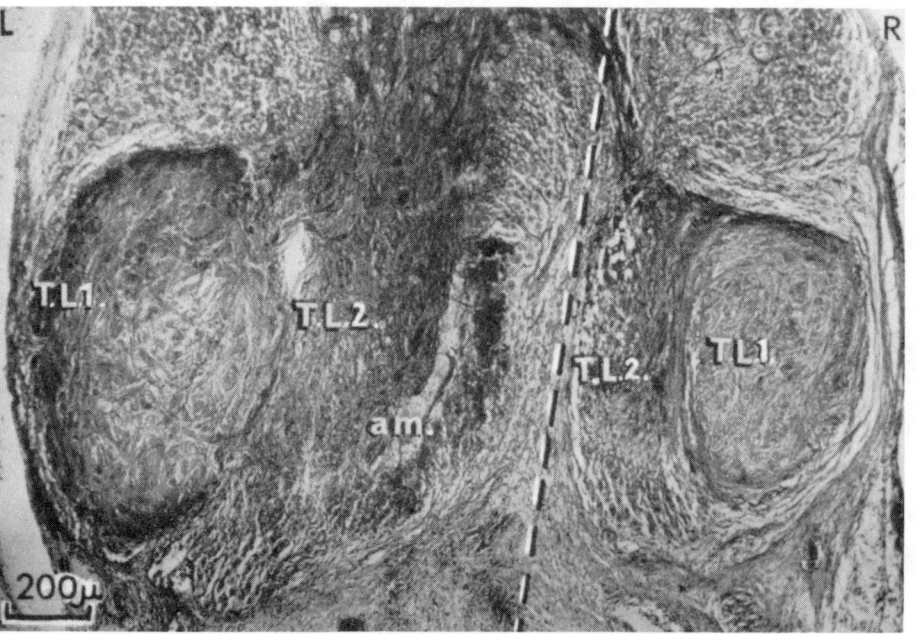

F<small>IG</small>. 24. Horizontal section of tactile learning centres of octopus after bisection. The cut has passed to the right of mid-line and has destroyed all small-celled tissue on that side. As a result, the left side was able to learn but not the right side (see fig. 25). am., amacrine cells. (Wells and Young, unpublished)

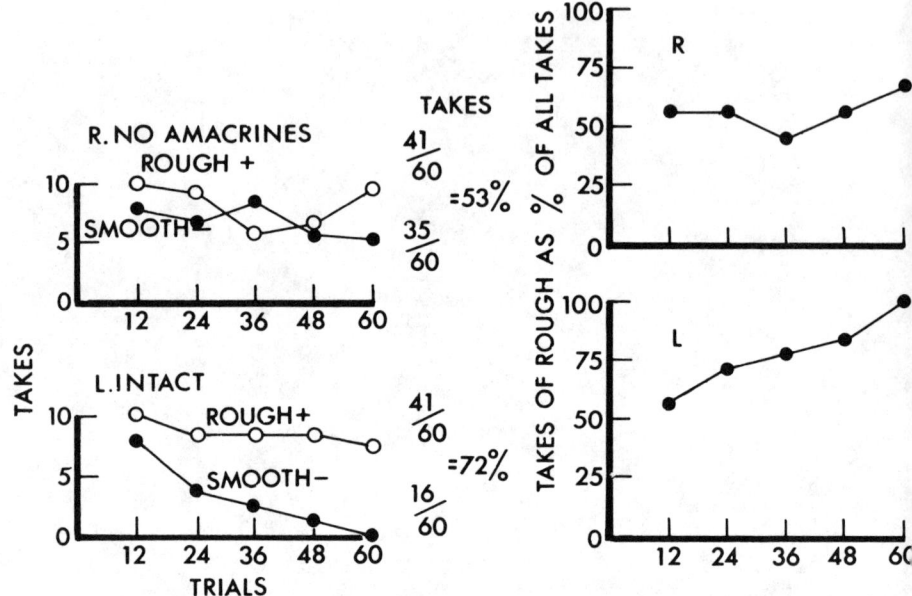

Fig. 25. Plot of sequence of learning by the preparation shown in fig. 24. Both sides were trained to take a rough cylinder (open circles) and reject a smooth one (solid circles). This was possible on left, but both cylinders continued to be drawn in on right. (Wells and Young, unpublished)

trometers on the relatively restricted regions that are concerned and to study whether the learning powers are affected by pharmacological agents, for example those that are are likely to inhibit protein synthesis.

There is certainly much work to be done. Even the gross details of the cells of this region are poorly known. A few of them have been seen stained with the Golgi method. Many of the large cells have two main trunks, and it is tempting to think of these as providing the two alternative pathways, for drawing in and for rejecting. But the sample available for study is small and imperfect. The small cells that send their axons into the neuropil alongside the large cells are packed with synaptic vesicles, like the similar cells of the vertical and subfrontal lobes (Graziadei, personal communication). They frequently show serial synapses, which provide the possible basis for presynaptic inhibition. If they have no long axon their function cannot be to transmit signals over a distance. It is much more likely that they serve to produce large amounts of a substance locally, perhaps the inhibitory transmitter. It is a problem why these cells are so small and numerous. It can hardly be to provide numerous specific channels. They must be highly redundant. Is it a matter of supplying large surface areas?

Unresolved Complications of the Hypothesis

In discussions of possible synaptic changes during learning it is usually assumed that the change is an increase in the ease of passage along a particular pathway, and that this increase occurs gradually, that is, partially on each occasion of learning (see, e.g., Taylor, 1964). The opposite hypotheses have been put forward here: that learning is by the inhibition of an unwanted pathway, and that this occurs suddenly and completely in each unit or module, the mnemon that is concerned. It would not fundamentally alter the character of the hypothesis to suppose that learning consists in lowering the threshold of the path that has been used. The circuits of figure 8 would be different in the sense that the collaterals would return to the pathway used, perhaps through small cells triggered to release material that increases excitability. There are various reasons for preferring the inhibitory hypothesis. The required negative feedback circuits are prominent in reflex systems and hence provide a ready-made system that with slight alteration could have evolved into a learning system. Positive feedback systems exist, but if they were used they would leave the alternative (unused) pathway still open (though unfacilitated) and in this sense the system would be inefficient. An even more serious difficulty is that the collateral system would have to increase the excitability of synapses in which they were not directly concerned (although made with the same cell). As Burns (1958) has pointed out, no such vicarious facilitation has ever been observed.[1] It is not impossible to imagine such a process,

---

[1] Heterosynaptic facilitation has however recently been recorded in a small proportion of neurons of the gastropod *Aplysia* (Kandel and Tauc, 1965).

for example by altering the level of polarisation of the whole cell, but the difficulty is less for the inhibitory hypothesis, especially if the clamp is placed by pre-synaptic inhibition.

However, the change may be in either direction or both. It is not even essential that there be more than one pathway. The alternative might be that the output from a given classifying cell be either used or not used. It is essential for the module to have classifying cells, each with one or more outputs, each provided with specialised systems capable of changing the probability of use of the channel after the arrival of impulses indicating the results of action.

The arrangement of the paired centres suggests that the signals of results are delivered in such a way as to compute the solution "attack—unless" for stimulation of each classifying cell. It is doubtful, however, whether this can be the complete solution. It does not allow for any direction of multiplied pain signals to the memory. No information is available as to types of combinations that are set up in the vertical lobe circuit. Are they all alike or are there various specific sorts? We are correspondingly ignorant in regard to the types of connection that are made in the feedback systems from the vertical (V.U.2) to the lateral superior frontal (V.L.1) and subvertical (V.L.2) to optic lobes. There may be much specificity, built-in or acquired, in these connections. If this is so, they may enter into the actual long-term storage functions of the memory in an even more intimate manner than has been suggested above.

It is assumed that the learning change is sudden and complete, for each cell concerned, on a single occasion of learning. This assumption is made because memory records of single occasions can be set up in men and animals, and rapid learning seems desirable for many situations in nature. However, there are obvious disadvantages as well as advantages in sudden changes in the probability of response. It is assumed here that changes in behaviour are not erratic because only some mnemons are switched at each occasion of learning. But it may well be that the learning cells are only partially switched at each "trial." This would again not fundamentally alter the hypothesis.

No provision is made here for erasure from the memory, since we have no evidence of this in the octopus. Human beings and animals certainly remember some things for a very long time. What we commonly call "forgetting" often seems to be more a matter of displacement by other "memories" or simply of failure to read-out from a record that is felt to be present though inaccessible. However, there might be a process of erasure, with re-use of units, although it is difficult to see how this would occur.

So many qualifications of the hypothesis must be made that in all honesty it must be admitted on examination to be little more than a rather vague guess. It is considered to be a guess worth making, however, not only to emphasise how little we know, but to direct attention to the nature of the information that we need.

The Evolution of the Learning Centres
of Cephalopods

The touch learning system of the octopus has special attraction in that it has arisen relatively recently in the course of evolution. It has provided us with strong hints as to how a system regulated only by the hereditary memory became converted into a system with the capacity to store information during its lifetime. The octopods probably diverged from the squids and the cuttlefishes at least one hundred million years ago, in the Cretaceous Period, perhaps earlier (Donovan, 1964). Both derived from a previous stock resembling the living *Nautilus.* The squids and other decapods have no elabourate touch memory system (fig. 21). These animals manœuvre under visual guidance and then shoot out the long arms to seize their prey. There is little or no tactile exploration of the object seized, which is immediately bitten. In *Octopus,* in contrast, the arms reach for a considerable distance and are continually used in exploration of situations that are out of sight. The arms thus operate as distance receptors. Learning which of the objects touched are likely to yield food must be of great importance. In *Nautilus* the supra-oesophageal or cerebral cord shows none of the special centres found in modern forms (Young, 1965 *b*), (fig. 26). Yet equivalent structures can be vaguely discerned, as if they are still only partly differentiated. The entire front of the cord is concerned with regulating the buccal mass. The rest of

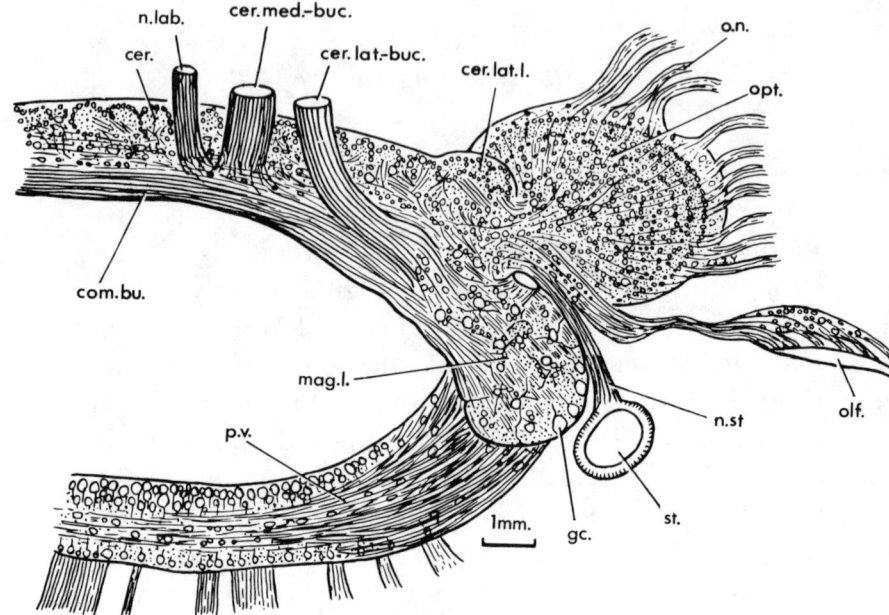

Fig. 26. Transverse section of circum-oesophageal nerve ring of primitive cephalopod, *Nautilus*. The simple eyes are presumably unable to report with accuracy on distant happenings. There is consequently relatively little development of the visual centres. The olfactory organ and its centres are large. The supra-oesophageal (cerebral) cord does not show the differentiated centres found in higher forms. It appears to be concerned mainly with control of eating and perhaps of bringing the animal to the situation where it can eat. cer., cerebral cord; cer. lat.-, cer. med.-buc., nerve trunks leading to ganglia that control the eating apparatus; cer.lat.1, lateral cerebral lobe; com. bu., commissural bundles; g. c., giant cell; mag.l., magnocellular lobe, a motor centre; n.lab., labial nerves; n.st., static nerves; olf., olfactory organ and nerve; opt., optic lobe; o.n., optic nerves; p.v., palliovisceral cord, a motor centre; st., statocyst, a gravity receptor. (Modified from Young, 1964a)

the cord provides systems that seem to allow oppor-
tunity for interaction between visual, tactile, and olfactory inputs. (The animal is macrosmatic and has a
pinhole camera eye.) There is no information on
whether the animal has a memory.

Perhaps the chief point to be learned from this
Nautilus brain is that the higher cerebral centres have
arisen within the system for the control of eating. Presumably a major part of the input from the special
receptors is concerned with getting the animal into a
situation where it can eat. In *Octopus* the touch memory system has developed out of the centre that at first
was concerned only with the control of the eating apparatus of the buccal mass and the correlation of this
control with that for arm movements.

Development of the Paired Centres of the Octopus

In an unhatched octopus the elaborate centres connected with the two memory systems have not yet
developed (fig. 27). The tactile system is a single
lobe in the position of the posterior buccal, hardly
distinguishable from the superior buccal lobe. The
median inferior frontal is a mere commissure in the
mid-line and the subfrontals are hardly apparent, as
groups of cells on the median wall (fig. 28). Thus
the small-celled special lobes develop above the basal
centres with large cells. The upper parts provide interweaving networks, and thus opportunities for interaction between inputs, and responses to particular sets
of them. The small cells of the upper parts, somehow
concerned with recording in the memory, are a devel-

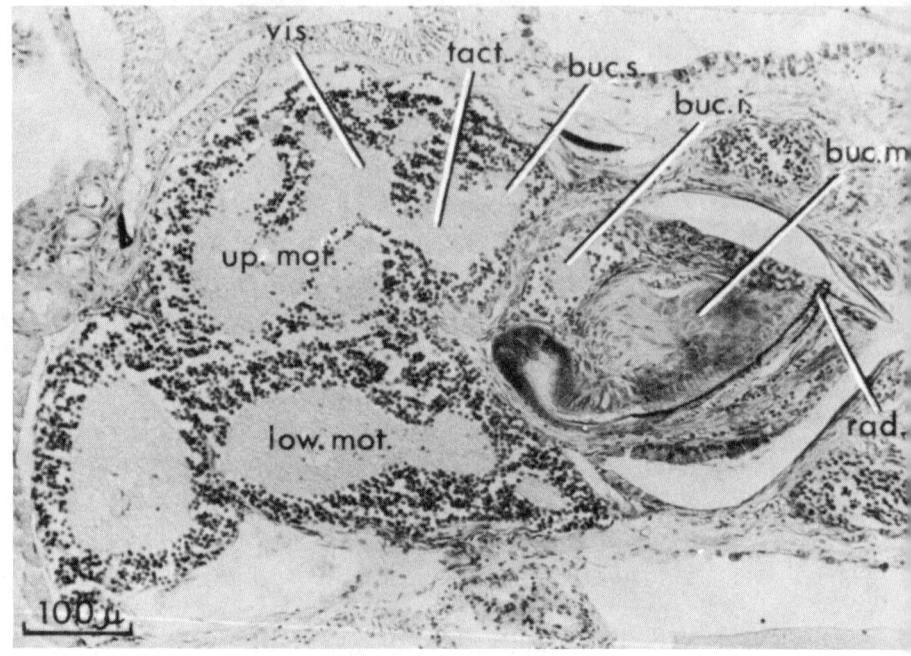

FIG. 27. Vertical longitudinal section through brain of a developing octopus. Note that lower centres are well developed before higher learning centres appear. buc.i., inferior buccal ganglion (centre for control of jaws and radula); buc.m., buccal mass, including muscles of jaws; buc.s., superior buccal ganglion, regulating all processes of killing and eating; low.mot., lower motor centres; rad., radula; tact., region where paired tactile centres will differentiate; at this stage they form a single lobe; up.mot., upper motor centres; vis., region where paired visual centres will differentiate; the median superior frontal and vertical lobes are just discernible at top. (Young, 1965c)

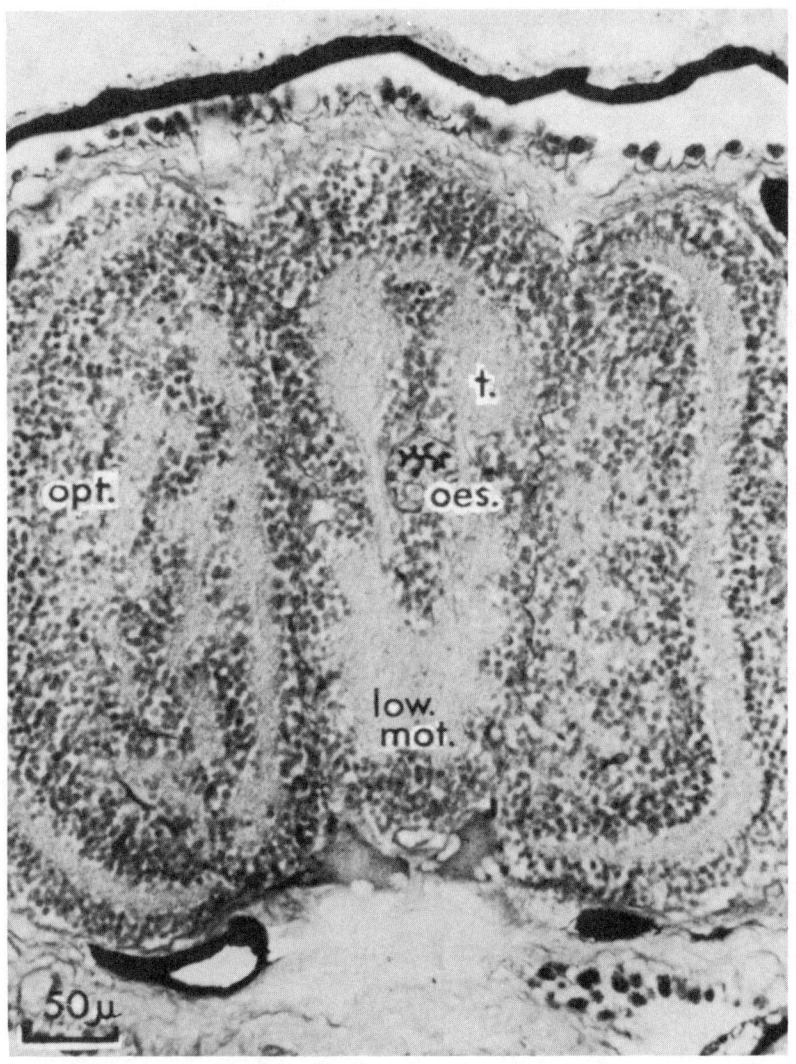

FIG. 28. Transverse section through unhatched octopus embryo at level of future paired tactile centres. At this stage they consist of a single pair of lobes (*t.*), joined by a commissure. The latter will develop into median inferior frontal lobe. low.mot., lower motor centres; oes., oesophagus; opt., optic lobe. (Young, 1965*c*)

opment of the small cells, mixed with the large, in the lower part of the system (fig. 29).

The visual memory centres also are hardly differentiated at the stage shown in figure 27. The subvertical lobe (second lower visual) is the centre out of which the others develop. It is broadly continuous with the second lower tactile centre (posterior buccal) (fig. 30). Thus the visual system, although much older than the tactile, probably developed originally by modification of the centres concerned with bringing the animal into a situation where it can eat.

These embryological facts may guide us in looking for the precursors of the memory systems. Learning cannot have appeared suddenly, but must have depended upon genetic changes that altered the previous synaptic arrangements, making them modifiable with use. Several workers have suggested that learning is based upon the alterations that take place in conduction through reflex arcs when they are either rested or strongly stimulated (see Eccles, 1964). The learning process must be a development of some such increase or decrease, with use, of conduction along pathways. The present hypothesis is that the chief factor is a decrease in the unwanted pathway, as by the continued release of an inhibitor.

The Origin of Learning

Even when the octopods were at a pre-memory stage, when seizure of food by the arms was the result of an inherited reflex mechanism, there must have been systems for inhibiting this seizure, for example at the

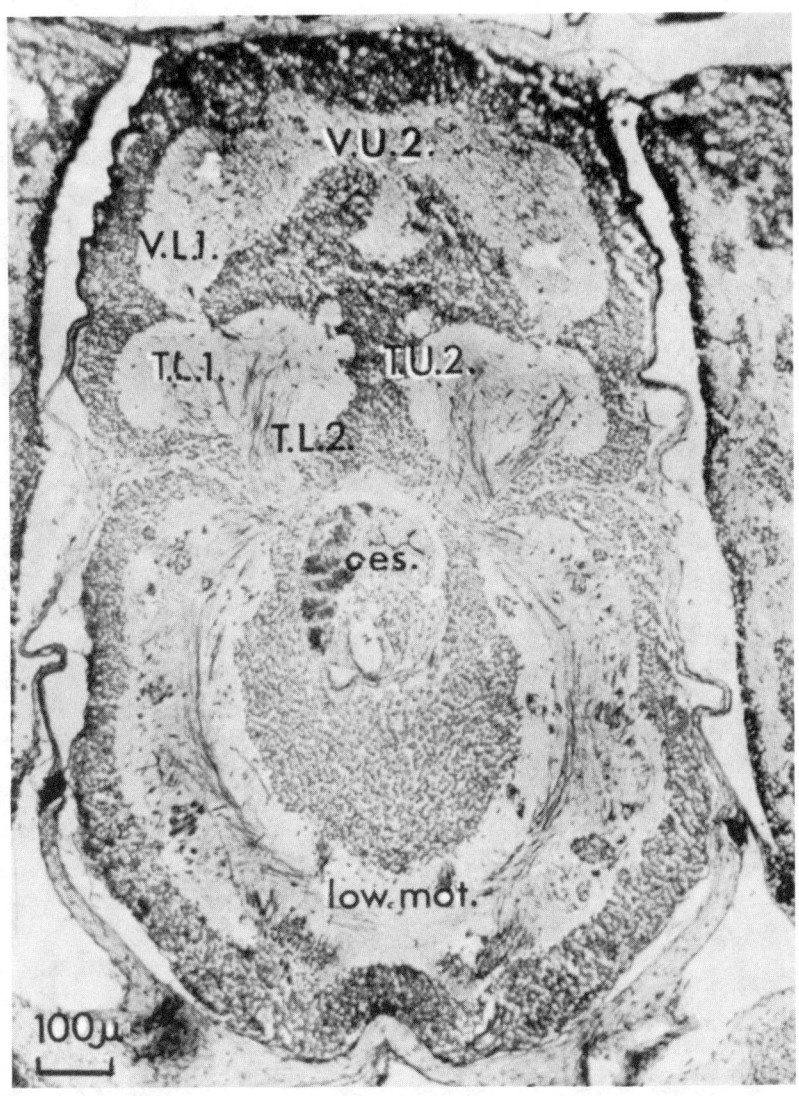

FIG. 29. Transverse section of front end of brain of an octopus at stage of hatching. The two lower tactile centres (T.L.1, T.L.2) are now differentiated. The second upper centre (T.U.2) is beginning to form as median wall of the original single lobe. The first upper centre does not show in this section. (Young, 1965c)

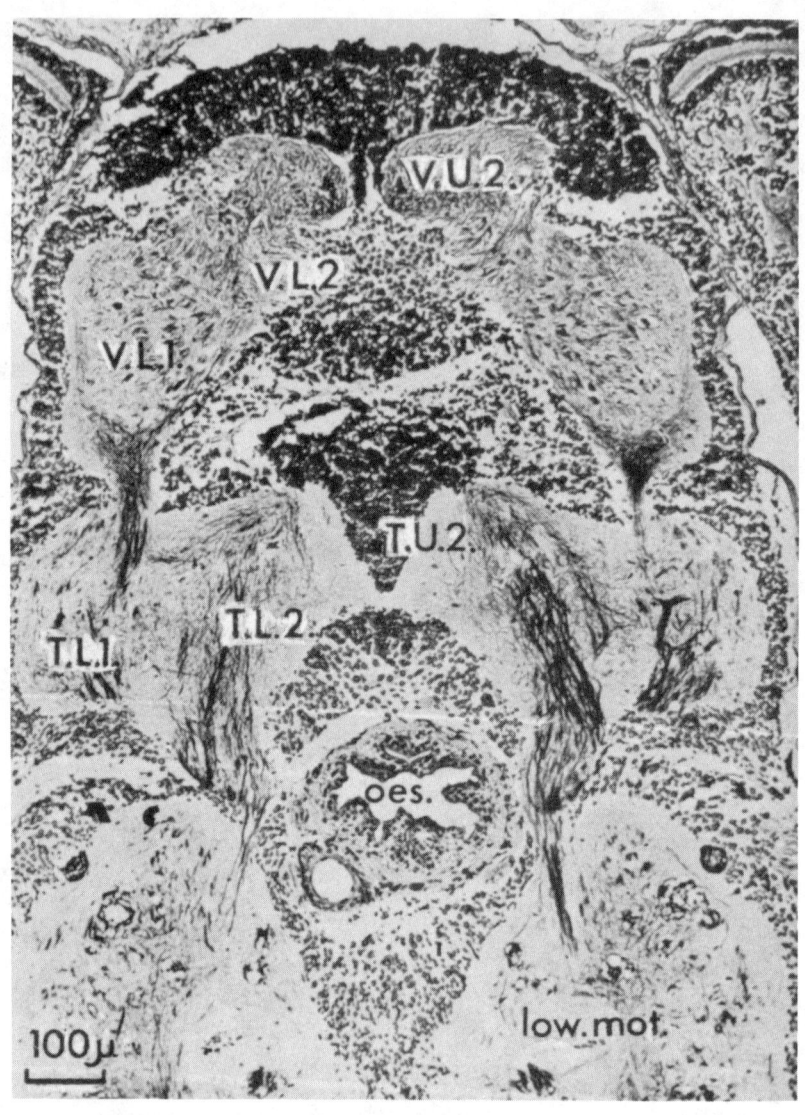

FIG. 30. Transverse section of front part of brain of a young octopus (2g). The tactile centres have further differentiated. Note that second upper centre (subfrontal) forms as median wall. The tactile first upper centre lies in another section. (Young, 1965c)

sudden onset of pain (figs. 31 and 32). In any animal organisation that permits a range of possible reflex actions there must be mechanisms for inhibiting the use of operations that are not required at the moment (Sherrington, 1947). This is an essential feature of the system of choices by which the homeostat operates. It is now suggested that the memory system has evolved by specialising the metabolism of the inhibitory cells so that they make long-lasting alterations in the probability of use of a given pathway. It has often been suspected that the basis of learning may be found in the changes that are known to occur during the use of reflex pathways, as in post-tetanic potentiation (Eccles and McIntyre, 1953). At first the change might have been simply a longer action of the inhibitory cells of certain reflex arcs, perhaps by eliminating responses that were consistently followed by pain. This would hardly be an efficient system to operate at the lowest motor levels if it led to the prolonged disuse of certain muscles. The development of alternative outputs at higher levels must have been an early stage in the evolution of the memory. The inhibitory systems, which already operated the hereditary mechanisms of choice, were then available with relatively little modification to close one channel and provide a long-lasting record. As evidence that something like this occurred, there are small cells in the superior buccal lobe, the reflex centre that controls eating in an octopus. Presumably they perform the function of inhibiting reflexes that are temporarily unwanted. The small cells lie mainly in the inner cell layers, near the neuropil. The centres for touch learning are directly continuous with this su-

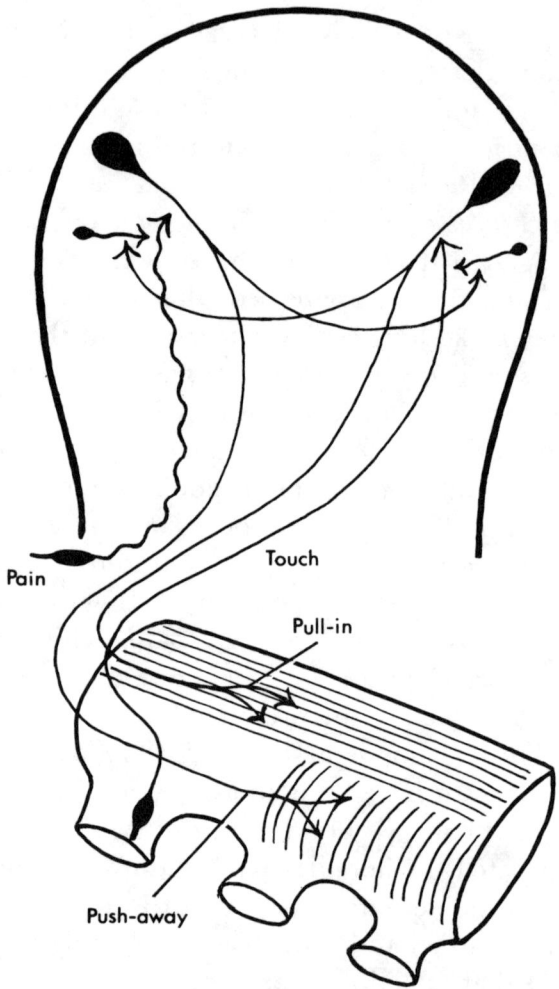

Fig. 31. Diagram of function of inhibitory small cells in a hypothetical purely reflex system. If sucker sense organ is stimulated alone, only one response, "pull-in," can occur. The opposite, "push-away," is inhibited by a collateral of the motor cell stimulating an inhibiting cell next to the cell controlling "push-away." Conversely, when pain receptors are stimulated, "push-away" is activated, "pull-in" inhibited.

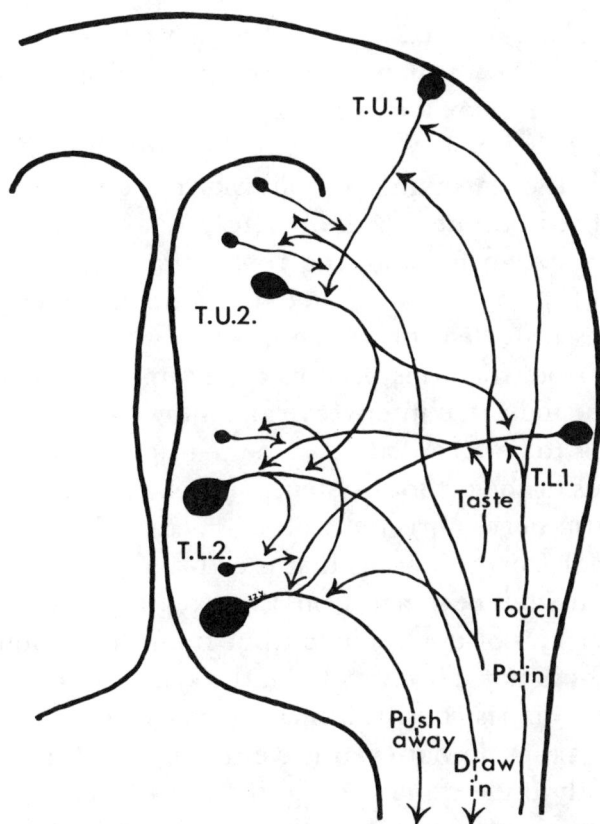

FIG. 32. Diagram of possible development of touch learning system from a reflex type as shown in fig. 31. The touch fibres have acquired two possible outputs through T.L.1. If, when a particular set of them is stimulated, "taste" results, the two sets of signals will combine in T.L.1 and activate the "draw in" neuron in T.L.2. This, through collaterals, will inhibit the "push-away" neuron in T.L.2. Inhibition can be set up by these two lobes acting alone, but is reinforced by the upper circuit through T.U.1 and T.U.2. The combination of touch and taste signals will reinforce the tendency to draw in (and inhibit the other) *unless* pain signals arrive, operating the "push-away" pathway.

perior buccal lobe, and their numerous minute cells are directly continuous with the inner layers of small cells in the reflex lobe (fig. 22).

Much is involved in making a useful learning system. If the classifying cells are not directly connected with fixed outputs it will obviously be advantageous to have a system for allowing representations of the actions of various sets of them to be set up in the memory. This is provided for in the octopus where the input fibres from the arms pass on to the upper part of the system, and there interweave and allow various combinations to be recorded. This is the origin of the upper circuits of the octopus systems. The significance of the fantastic nerve-fibre webs of the median inferior and superior frontal lobes is that they make possible many combinations of signals from the receptors and of those with signals of taste. The output from these combinations does not, however, leave the system at once, but passes to lobes consisting mainly of still smaller cells, whose axons do not even leave the lobe. While we do not fully understand the significance of these minute cells, the evidence is that they allow signals of pain to establish, when necessary, their effects in the memory. Both taste and pain signals were already entering the pre-memory system, serving to operate the appropriate reflexes. To produce a memory system, the specific afferents and the fibres carrying signals of results have continued into literally "higher" regions, above the reflex ones. These regions contain small and very small cells, which operate upon the combined inputs and then return signals to the more basal regions, where the actual memory cells lie. These may be relatively large cells with alternative possible outlets, one of which is then closed.

This sequence of changes has been discussed in relation to the touch learning system because this is a relatively recent acquisition and it has been possible to suggest how it may have arisen. The visual centres probably had a similar origin, much earlier. Their output is through the second lower centre, the subvertical lobe, which is a direct backward continuation of the posterior buccal lobe. The optic lobe can be regarded as an immense outgrowth of the subvertical. It appears clearly in *Nautilus* as a lateral extension of the supra-oesophageal cord (fig. 26). The optic system, like the tactile, has grown out of the feeding system. All cephalopods, being carnivores, depend upon making correct predictions about the probability of obtaining food from objects attacked from a distance or touched. To make such predictions it has been an advantage to them to develop a neural memory system, which provides instructions that can be brought up to date more rapidly than is possible by the hereditary mechanism alone.

The touch learning system, acquired relatively recently by octopods, has been lost again in some members of that order. The Argonautidae are octopuses that have left the sea bottom and returned to live at the sea surface. In them the whole inferior frontal system has become greatly reduced, presumably because the information from the arms is of less value for life away from the bottom.

Control of the Collection of Information

The means for collecting information presumably change continually as organisms evolve. Nature thus develops a series of mechanisms, each suitable for dealing with a particular environment. To study the functioning of these variants of nervous organisation is the true comparative neurology. Such study requires that we understand the evolutionary history of the types of animal concerned. The variants that are revealed help to show the fundamental modes of functioning of the nervous system.

One of the most interesting variables among animal species is the length of life between generations. There is obviously some relation between the acquiring of information by shuffling the genetic determinants and the more direct means provided by the nervous system. There are enormous differences in length of life. A bacterium may live for ten minutes, a protozoan for some days (say 10^3 mins). Many animals live for a year $(5 \times 10^5$ mins), larger ones for several years (up to 10^7 mins), and very few for 10^8, which is about a hundred years. What is the significance of these differences of one hundred million times in lengths of life? Surely it is that bacteria can live in only a limited range of habitats, in spite of their adaptability, whereas large organisms have more elaborate homeostatic equipment and take longer to unfold it. This is one of the distinctions we have in mind when we say that mammals are higher organisms than bacteria (Young, 1962 *a*).

The size of the brain and the length of life are

clearly related. Mammals with small brains breed often, and vice versa. The relationship is not precise, perhaps because we do not know how to measure the nervous system. To weigh it or even to count its cells is but a crude procedure. But clearly there is some relationship between brain and length of life and it is interesting that in a wide variety of animals the length of life is itself regulated by nerve centres that lie close to the learning mechanism, or are even a part of it. In mammals the rate of maturation is controlled by the hypothalamus, through the pituitary. The hypothalamo-hypophyseal tract is the only motor nerve leaving the forebrain and, incidentally, it works by neurosecretion.

Similar arrangements control the development of insects and crustacea and we have now found essentially the same arrangement in cephalopods. The optic gland controls the time of maturity of the female octopus and is itself controlled by a nerve arising from a centre immediately below the learning centres (Boycott and Young, 1955; Wells and Wells, 1959). It is not known that neurosecretion is involved here.

The Human Information-Collecting System

This similar situation in phyla so diverse is one of many instances in which similar problems evoke similar mechanisms. As animals evolved better powers of learning, it was necessary to find means of ensuring that they lived long enough to learn. As we come to see more precisely how such mechanisms play a part in the homeostasis of the species we shall know better what significant features of the control system to look for.

This may be of especial importance to Man, in whom the mechanism for acquiring information by the individual is greatly hypertrophied, and the time of development and maturation correspondingly lengthened. The acceleration of the rate of change in man's condition over the last few millennia has been the result of the development of codes by which information can be passed directly from one individual to another. This might be called "multiparental inheritance." We acquire information not just from two parents but from many. Indeed, we establish artificial information stores outside our bodies. We thus, as it were, construct models of the world outside our brains and outside our own genetic system. By proper use of these models we should be able to elaborate a system of homeostasis that overcomes all the risks posed by the environment.

But obviously there are dangers of misusing these powers. There must be co-operation between individuals and this means training during a prolonged pre-adult period. Only by delay in the development of fully adult characters do individuals become sufficiently tractable to operate the powerful systems that have developed. It has been said that man is a foetal ape. To paraphrase this—we are men because we never reach full apehood. To continue to develop our capacities for co-operation is perhaps the chief task confronting mankind. We must become even more like little children. The basis of this change may well be neurendocrine systems such as those we have been discussing. To find the principles upon which maturation is regulated in diverse animals may provide a modest contribution to man's survival.

References

Adey, W. R., C. W. Dunlop, and C. E. Hendrix
    1960   Hippocampal slow waves. Distribution and phase relationships in the course of approach learning. *Arch. Neurol., 3*: 74-90.

Aitken, J. T., and J. E. Bridger
    1961   Neuron size and neuron population density in the lumbosacral region of the cat's spinal cord. *J. Anat. (Lond.) 95*: 38-53.

Bitterman, M. E.
    1965   The evolution of intelligence. *Sci. Amer., 212*: 92-100.

Boycott, B. B., and J. Z. Young
    1950   The comparative study of learning. *Symp. Soc. Exp. Biol., 4*: 432-453.
    1955   Memories controlling attacks on food objects by *Octopus vulgaris* Lamarck. *Pubbl. Staz. Zool. Napoli, 27*: 232-249.

Burns, B. D.
    1958   *The Mammalian Cerebral Cortex.* London: Edward Arnold (Publishers) Ltd.

Burrows, T., I. Campbell, E. Howe, and J. Z. Young
    1965   Conduction, velocity and diameter of nerve fibres of cephalopods. *J. Physiol. (Lond.), 179*: 39-40.

Cannon, W. B.
    1932   *The Wisdom of the Body.* New York: W. W. Norton.

Cherkin, A.
    1966   *Proc. Nat. Acad. Sci., 55*, January 1966.

Colonnier, M.
    1964   The tangential organisation of the visual cortex.
           J. Anat. (Lond.), *98*: 327-344.
Craik, K. J. W.
    1943   *The Nature of Explanation.* Cambridge University
           Press.
Deutsch, J. A.
    1960*a* The plexiform zone and shape recognition in the
           octopus. *Nature (Lond.)*, *185*: 443-446.
    1960*b* Theories of shape discrimination in *Octopus. Na-
           ture (Lond.)*, *188*: 1090-1092.
Dilly, P. N.
    1963   Delayed responses in *Octopus. J. Exp. Biol., 40*: 393-
           401.
Dodwell, P. C.
    1957   Shape discrimination in the octopus and the rat.
           Nature (Lond.), *179*: 1088.
    1961   Facts and theories of shape discrimination. *Nature
           (Lond.)*, *191*: 578-581.
Donovan, D. J.
    1964   Cephalopod phylogeny and classification. *Biol.
           Rev., 39*: 259-287.
Eccles, J. C.
    1964   *The Physiology of the Synapse.* Berlin: Springer-
           Verlag.
Eccles, J. C., and A. K. McIntyre
    1953   The effects of disuse and activity on mammalian
           spinal reflexes. *J. Physiol. (Lond.)*, *121*: 492-516.
Gaze, R. M.
    1960   Regeneration of the optic nerve in Amphibia. *Int.
           Rev. Neurobiol., 2*: 1-40.
Gray, E. G.
    1962   A morphological basis for pre-synaptic inhibition?
           Nature (Lond.), *193*: 82-83.
    1964   Tissue of the central nervous system. In *Electron
           Microscopic Anatomy*, ed. S. M. Kurtz. New York:
           Academic Press.

Gray, E. G., and J. Z. Young
    1964   Electron microscopy of the synaptic structure of *Octopus* brain. *J. Cell. Biol.*, *21*: 87-103.

Hubel, D. H., and T. N. Wiesel
    1959   Receptive fields of single neurons in the cat's striate cortex. *J. Physiol. (Lond.)*, *148*: 574-591.
    1962   Receptive fields, binocular interaction and functional architecture in the cat's visual cortex. *J. Physiol. (Lond.)*, *160*: 106-154.
    1963   Shape and arrangement of columns in cat's striate cortex. *J. Physiol. (Lond.)*, *165*: 559-568.
    1965   Receptive fields and functional architecture in two nonstriate visual areas (18 and 19) of the cat. *J. Neurophysiol.*, *28*: 229-289.

Hydén, H.
    1960   The neuron, in *The Cell*, vol. 4, eds. J. Brachet and A. E. Mirsky. New York and London: Academic Press, 216-308.

Jasper, H. H., C. F. Ricci, and B. Doane
    1958   Patterns of cortical neuronal discharge during conditioned responses in monkeys. In *Ciba Foundation Symposium. Neurological Bases of Behaviour*, eds. G. E. W. Wolstenholme and C. M. O'Connor. London: Churchill.

Jasper, H. H., and G. D. Smirnov (eds.)
    1960   Moscow colloquium in electroencephalography of higher nervous activity. *E.E.G. Journal (Montreal)*.

Kandel, E. R., and L. Tauc
    1965   Heterosynaptic facilitation in neurones of the abdominal ganglion of *Aplysia depilans*. *J. Physiol. (Lond.)*, *181*: 1-27.

Kidd, M.
    1962   Electron microscopy of the inner plexiform layer of the retina in the cat and the pigeon. *J. Anat. (Lond.)*, *96*: 179-187.

Kuffler, S. W., and D. D. Potter
    1964   Glia in the leech central nervous system—physio-

logical properties and neuron-glia relationships. *J. Neurophysiol.*, *27*: 290-320.

Lorente de Nó, R.
    1936   Responses of oculomotor nucleus, facilitation and delay paths. *Amer. J. Physiol.*, *112*: 595-609.

Mackintosh, J.
    1962   An investigation of reversal learning in *Octopus vulgaris* Lamarck. *Quart. J. Exp. Psychol.*, *14*: 15-22.

Mackintosh, N. J., and J. Mackintosh
    1964*a*   The effect of overtraining on a nonreversal shift in *Octopus. J. Gen. Psychol.*, *106*: 373-377.
    1964*b*   Performance of *Octopus* over a series of reversals of a simultaneous discrimination. *Anim. Behav.*, *12*: 321-324.

Maldonado, H.
    1963*a*   The positive learning process in *Octopus vulgaris. Z. vergl. Physiol.*, *47*: 191-214.
    1963*b*   The general amplification function of the vertical lobe in *Octopus vulgaris. Z. vergl. Physiol.*, *47*: 215-229.
    1963*c*   The control of attack by *Octopus. Z. vergl. Physiol.*, *47*: 656-674.
    1963*d*   The visual attack learning system in *Octopus vulgaris. J. Theoret. Biol.*, *5*: 470-488.
    1965   Positive and negative learning processes in *Octopus vulgaris* and the effect of the removal of the vertical and median superior frontal lobes. *Z. vergl. Physiol.* (In press.)

Messenger, J. B.
    1963   Behaviour of young *Octopus briareus* Robson. *Nature (Lond.)*, *197*: 1186-1187.

Morrell, F.
    1960   Microelectrode and steady potential studies suggesting a dendritic locus of closure. In Moscow colloquium in electroencephalography of higher nervous activity, eds. H. H. Jasper and G. D. Smirnov. *E.E.G. Journal (Montreal)*.

1961 Electrophysiological contributions to the neural basis of learning. *Physiol. Rev.*, *41*: 443-494.

Mountcastle, V. B.
1957 Modality and topographic properties of single neurons of cat's striate cortex. *J. Neurophysiol.*, *20*: 408-434.

Muntz, W. R. A.
1961 Interocular transfer in *Octopus vulgaris*. *J. Comp. Physiol. Psychol.*, *54*: 49-55.

Muntz, W. R. A., N. S. Sutherland, and J. Z. Young
1962 Simultaneous shape discrimination in *Octopus* after removal of the vertical lobe. *J. Exp. Biol.*, *39*: 557-566.

Neumann, J. von
1958 *The Computer and the Brain.* Silliman Memorial Lectures. New Haven: Yale University Press.

Nixon, M.
1966 Food intake and weight increase in *Octopus vulgaris*. (In preparation.)

Parriss, J. R., and J. Z. Young
1962 The limits of transfer of a learned discrimination to figures of larger and smaller sizes. *Z. vergl. Physiol.*, *45*: 618-635.

Penfield, W., and L. Roberts
1959 *Speech and Brain-mechanisms.* London: Oxford University Press.

Powell, T. P. S., and V. B. Mountcastle
1959 Some aspects of the functional organisation of the cortex of the postcentral gyrus of the monkey: a correlation of findings obtained in a single unit analysis with cytoarchitecture. *Johns Hopkins Hosp. Bull.*, *105*: 1333-162.

Sanders, F. K., and J. Z. Young
1940 Learning and other functions of the higher nervous centres of *Sepia*. *J. Neurophysiol.*, *3*: 501-526.

Sherrington, C. S.
1947 *The Integrative Action of the Nervous System*, rev. ed. New Haven: Yale University Press, 1961.

Sholl, D. A.
 1956 *The Organisation of the Cerebral Cortex*. London: Methuen.
Sommerhoff, G.
 1950 *Analytical Biology*. London: Oxford University Press.
Sutherland, N. S.
 1957 Visual discrimination of orientation and shape by the octopus. *Nature (Lond.)*, *179*: 11-13.
 1963 Shape discrimination and receptive fields. *Nature (Lond.)*, *197*: 118-122.
Sutherland, N. S., and J. Mackintosh
 1964 Discrimination learning: Non-additivity of cues. *Nature (Lond.)*, *201*: 528-530.
Taylor, W. K.
 1964 Cortico-thalamic organisation and memory. *Proc. Roy. Soc. B*, *159*: 466-478.
Wall, P. D.
 1964 Presynaptic control of impulses at the first central synapse in the cutaneous pathway. *Prog. in Brain Res.*, 12.
Wells, M. J.
 1960 Proprioception and visual discrimination of orientation in *Octopus*. *J. Exp. Biol.*, *37*: 489-499.
 1961 Centres for tactile and visual learning in the brain of *Octopus*. *J. Exp. Biol.*, *38*: 811-826.
Wells, M. J., and J. Wells
 1957 The effect of lesions to the vertical and optic lobes on tactile discrimination in *Octopus*. *J. Exp. Biol.*, *34*: 378-393.
 1959 Hormonal control of sexual maturity in *Octopus*. *J. Exp. Biol.*, *36*: 1-33.
Welsh, J. H.
 1961 Neuro hormones of Mollusca. *Amer. Zool.*, *1*: 267-272.
Wyckoff, R. W. G., and J. Z. Young
 1956 The motorneuron surface. *Proc. Roy. Soc. B*, *144*: 440-450.

Young, J. Z.

1938   The evolution of the nervous system and of the relationship of organism and environment. In *Evolution. Essays Presented to E. S. Goodrich*, ed. G. R. de Beer. Oxford: Clarendon Press.

1958   Effect of removal of various amounts of the vertical lobes on visual discrimination by *Octopus*. *Proc. Roy. Soc. B, 149*: 463-483.

1960*a*   The visual system of *Octopus*. 1. Regularities in the retina and optic lobes of *Octopus* in relation to form discrimination. *Nature (Lond.), 186*: 836-839.

1960*b*   The failures of discrimination learning following removal of the vertical lobes in *Octopus*. *Proc. Roy. Soc. B, 153*: 18-46.

1962*a*   *The Life of Vertebrates*, 2d ed. Oxford: Clarendon Press.

1962*b*   The optic lobes of *Octopus vulgaris*. *Phil. Trans. Roy. Soc. B, 245*: 19-58.

1962*c*   Why do we have two brains? Paper read at Conference on Cerebral Dominance, Johns Hopkins University School of Medicine, Baltimore, Md., April 23-25, 1961.

1963*a*   The number and sizes of nerve cells in *Octopus*. *Proc. Zool. Soc. Lond., 140*: Pt 2, 229-254.

1963*b*   Some essentials of neural memory systems. Paired centres that regulate and address the signals of the results of action. *Nature (Lond.), 198*: 626-630.

1964*a*   *A Model of the Brain*. Oxford: Clarendon Press.

1964*b*   Paired centres for the control of attack by *Octopus*. *Proc. Roy. Soc. B, 159*: 565-588.

1965*a*   The organisation of a memory system. Croonian Lecture of the Royal Society, delivered on May 6, 1965. *Proc. Roy. Soc. B, 163*: 285-320.

1965*b*   The central nervous system of *Nautilus*. *Phil. Trans. Roy. Soc. B, 249*: 1-25.

1965*c*   The centres for touch discrimination in *Octopus vulgaris*. *Phil. Trans. Roy. Soc. B, 249*: 45-67.

Index